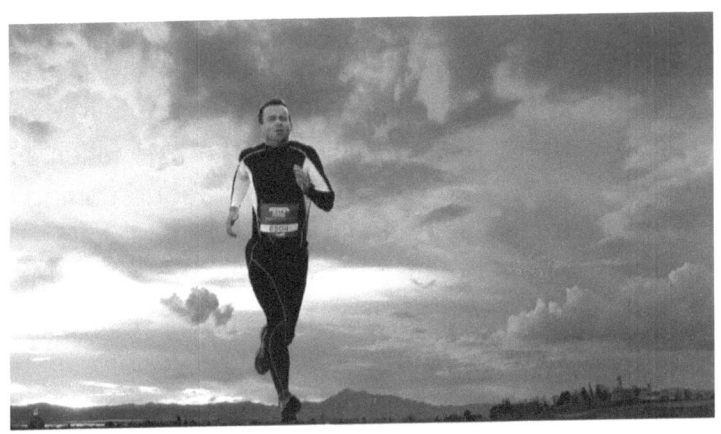

RUNNING AMERICA

A HALF MARATHON DIARY

By

FIFTY STATE RUNNER

Copyright © 2018

YouTube "Fifty State Runner Reprise"

(https://youtu.be/LTtgitm04no)

INTRODUCTION

This book is a multimedia diary describing an unexpected half marathon journey through every state in America. I haven't always been a runner, it's certainly not in my genetics. Now as I near the end of the road I find that I feel about running like Ralph Waldo Emerson felt about books when he said, "I cannot remember the books I've read any more than the meals I have eaten; even so, they have made me." So here's to all the runners out there who may not be super-fast, but share a passion for an old pair of running shoes and the open road. Remember, you don't have to be born to run to run for life.

So what's in this book? This book contains video links that visually document each race (usually about 2-4 minutes each in length), the printed video transcript, and the actual social-media lead-in to each state that I posted at the time of the race. Thus, the content has a very informal, impromptu and unrehearsed feel to it. My hope in this book is to authentically preserve the real-time journey, as it happened.

Before we get started, you should know the real reasons I started running. First, my teenage son and I had struggled with weight issues for many years. My wife and I often talked about what we could do to help our son lose weight. We decided that I would set the example by counting calories and intensifying my exercise regimen. Our secret evil plan was to have our son see results in me and decide to join the program. To my (and especially my son's) shock and awe, the pounds were falling off me in bunches. My son decided, on his own, to follow his dad's example. In six months I had lost over 70 pounds, and my son had lost 75 pounds. Our plan worked.

Second, I was at a point in my life where I really needed a goal. At that point, I had run in several events in Utah and Wyoming (including several half marathons, two full marathons, and one ultra). It occurred to me to set a goal to eventually run in every state. In hindsight, it has been a tremendous motivational activity for me, my family, and my friends.

I decided on half marathons because running every state felt like a big goal and I'd have to be ready at any moment to go the distance. Most of the races were targets of opportunity (i.e., not pre-planned). The most intense week was five states in eight days. Two other times I did four states in eight days. The others were mostly one at a time. As far as training, for the last many years my schedule has been 9 miles Monday and Wednesday and 15 miles on Saturday. I love running. I tell people it's my downtime.

Every race was a unique puzzle piece to the richness of the whole experience. That said, Maine, Pennsylvania, Delaware, and Oregon were especially emotional for me. Maine because it was the first time I had done two events in two days. Pennsylvania because I broke a PR that had stood for 25 states. Delaware because it was my last race on the Atlantic coastline and last state east of the Mississippi. Oregon because it was my last. Some of the most beautiful included Michigan's Grand Island in Lake Superior, Washington's Olympic Mountains, Alaska's Santa Claus run in North Pole, South Dakota's Deadwood Mickelson Trail, and Oregon's Sunset Bay. The very best moments and races were the ones that my wife was with me. We experienced 21 of the 50 states together, and she ran the 5K in many of those events.

One final note; I've learned through compiling this book that video transcription, even when transcribed by hand, doesn't always result in entirely coherent sentence structure. Please forgive this reality.

Table of Contents

LEGAL NOTES

UT TOP OF UTAH HALF
The Beehive State

First Half Marathon
(220 lbs)

Three Years Later
(150 lbs)

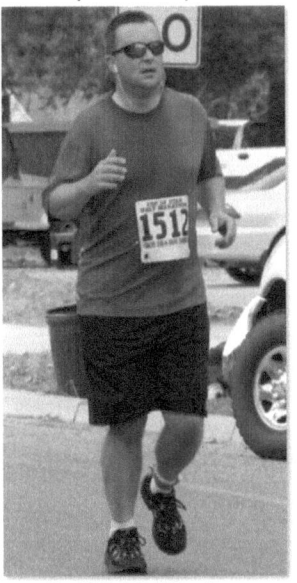

Top Of Utah Half Marathon

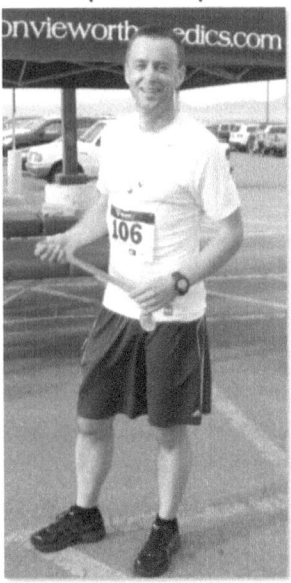

Smithfield Half Marathon

SOCIAL MEDIA NOTE

A few years ago, I lost 70 pounds, mostly by running (yup, sorry guys ... the answer is diet and exercise). I also ran a few marathons and a 50k ultra in the process. Finally, I set a goal to run a half marathon in all 50 states. Well, here's Utah. Enjoy!

VIDEO TRANSCRIPT

It was the start of a new year, and my daughter's December wedding had blown my racing-bicycle budget. I needed a new goal. It was then that I decided to run a half-marathon in every state.

Before I start glorifying my half-marathon runs, I need to give homage to my longest race. It was a crisp October morning many years ago when I ran 32 miles in Goblin Valley. I slept in my van in Green River the night before and then drove to Goblin Valley. It was a great experience, but I often wonder what inspired this crazy video…

> *Here I am on October 26. I've arrived under cover of darkness in the valley of the Goblins. I'm here to run thirty-two miles. …What was that? Just kidding. … I need to do something different today than I did four weeks ago when I ran a marathon. After 13 miles I wondered what I was thinking, and after 20 I stopped thinking at all. I limped through on muscles that were spasming. So today I'm going to do something different. I'm going to run a little slower, and I'm going to eat and drink a lot more. Now, I understand that I might be able to make it a little better if I could get some goblin meat. So that's my goal. If I see a goblin, I'm running after that guy. I'm going to tackle it, and I'm going to eat him. We'll see how I do. See ya. Bye.*

> *Now I'm coming up on the 16-mile mark and turn around point. My legs feel like they've gone 16 miles. It didn't help, at mile eight; we were, two of us, attacked by three goblins. One of them was huge, so naturally, I went after him. I caught his leg and tackled him, shoestring tackle sort of thing. Then he got up, and he could run faster than me by the time I reached mile eight, so I couldn't catch him. I went back and helped him get the other two, we ate those guys. Um, so that was ok, but still, I'm in need of some serious*

nourishment. So, I'm looking forward to the turn-around point when I can come back, and maybe I can get that guy … but they're all around us. I think they're just leaving me alone because I'm so awesome. Anyway, I'll talk to you at the end.

That was like the hardest thing I have ever done in my life. And it didn't help that around mile 22 that goblin came back! I was running away because I was really tired, but it was attacking someone. I was just going to go on, but it was a girl. So, I decided that I'd go back. So, I go and tackle this guy. He bit my ankle and for like the last eight miles or so my ankle was bleeding. That's the worst. So anyway, I finally drag him for a while until he dies and then I just put him over my shoulder and brought him here to the end. I think we're going to eat him. So anyway, thirty-two miles at the finish here at Goblin Valley. We'll see you later.

Like the Goblin Valley Ultra, I need to mention my two full marathons. Top of Utah the year before Goblin Valley and the Huntsville marathon a little more than a year later.

Before I had decided to run in each state, I had finished six half-marathons, two marathons, and one Ultra all in Utah. One of my favorites was the Provo midnight half marathon because my son ran it with me. My wife ran several with me including the Layton Half. My first race was the Top of Utah half marathon right here in cache valley (I was 70 pounds heavier then). I wouldn't run in another official event for three more years. Shortly after that, half marathon candidates suddenly opened up to all the states.

https://youtu.be/HOOym9cSBHA

WY Star Valley Half

The Equality State

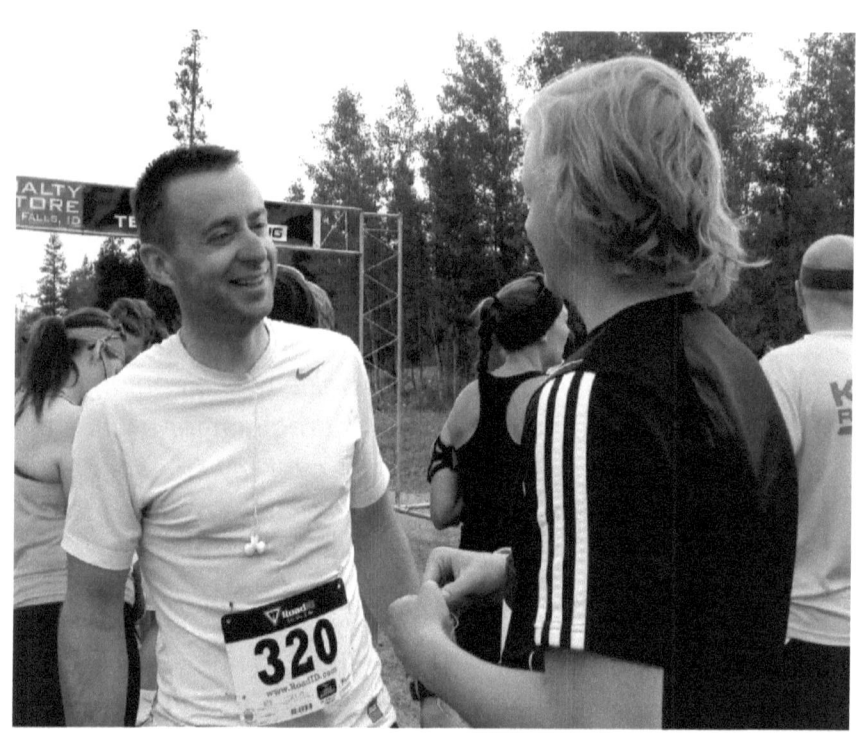

Social Media Note

Home to Yellowstone, Devils Tower, and my parent's childhood. Wyoming has always been a second home for me, so It seems fitting that it was state #2 in my half marathon quest. I can tell you that the Star Valley half marathon route is among the most beautiful garden spots on the earth. I'll definitely be back!

Video Transcript

Wyoming was the only state, other than Utah that I ran before my goal to run in every state. It is also a handful of states without any video ... sorry about that! After running a third of the states at this recording, Wyoming remains my second fastest time next to the Kentucky Derby half. Again, I was happy to have my son at my side on this race. He and I ran this race while at a reunion at the family farmhouse in Afton. Awesome huh. Wyoming ... Check!

https://youtu.be/NOnFLXrN-_U

CA The Hollywood Half
The Golden State

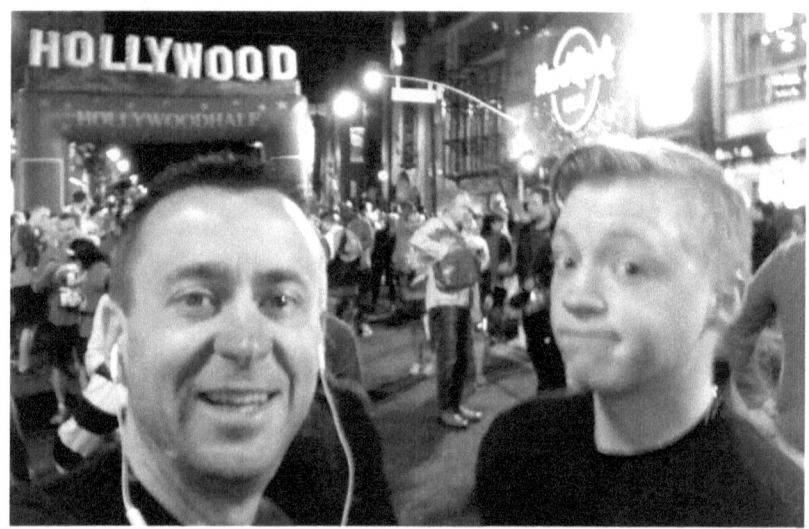

Social Media Note

Sun, beaches, and dolphin cruises, here's #3 ... California! Note that California was the first of four consecutive half-marathons in four states in four weeks ... it makes me tired just thinking about it ;). Cheers!

Video Transcript

California was #3. I still remember that my son and I got up early the morning of the race and walked the four blocks to the starting line on Hollywood and Highland. As we approached, I was amazed how many people were converging on the intersection. Just before the gun, we separated into our assigned corrals. The gun sounded, and we were off. We spent the most time on Hollywood Boulevard but also ran on

Highland Ave, Santa Monica Blvd, and others. I saw my son only once as I headed back to the finish (it was an out and back). After the race, we walked back to the hotel noting all the names etched into the stars on the sidewalk. Incidentally, my wife was also signed up for this race, but the month before the race she broke her ankle and tore a tendon which required surgery, so she didn't get to run. My youngest son was also with us. During the time we weren't racing, we stopped in Las Vegas, watched the Bellagio fountains, spent time on the California beaches (where my son dug a hole as tall as himself), and enjoyed a dolphin watching cruise. This is the last race my son has run with me so far, but I'm sure he'll join me on another one soon.

https://youtu.be/aRkvzAM_GUo

FL PENSACOLA BEACH HALF

The Sunshine State

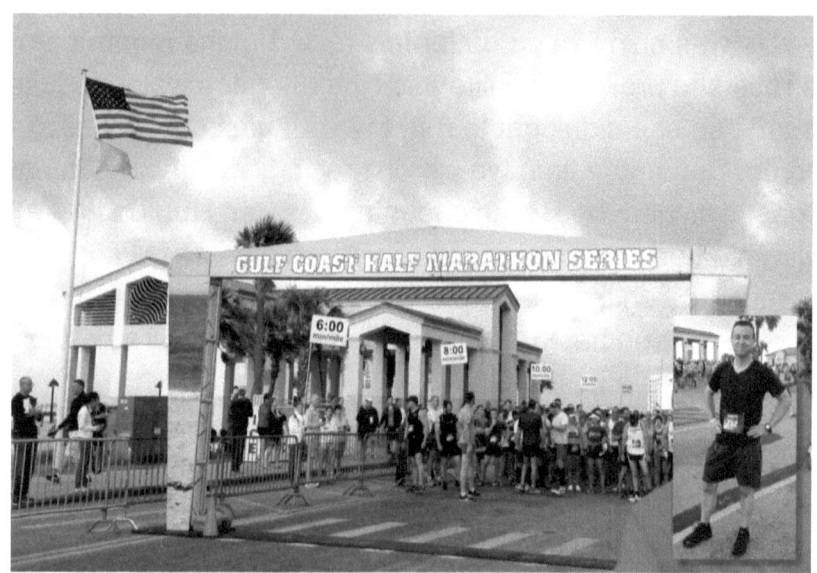

SOCIAL MEDIA NOTE

What's your favorite US public beach? I've been to quite a few US beaches, and if you are into fun, non-lonely stretches of sand, then the Emerald Coast and Pensacola Beach gets my vote. Here's state #4 ... Florida! My lovely wife accompanied me in Florida, and we had a fantastic time riding a dinner/theater train, visiting the sites, and frequenting the beach!

VIDEO TRANSCRIPT

I've visited many of America's coastlines, and I must say Pensacola hosts one of my favorite public beaches. It has plenty of activity and a terrific atmosphere without feeling too crowded. It was great to have my wife with me on this one. We rode the Seminole Gulf Railway murder mystery train, and my wife won the "Super Sleuth" award by most correctly solving this mysterious who-done-it performance on a moving train. We also had a fun caricature drawing done of us as. The entire Half Marathon was on Pensacola beach in a perfect ocean breeze.

https://youtu.be/Jp06qCtCNAQ

KY Kentucky Derby Mini

The Bluegrass State

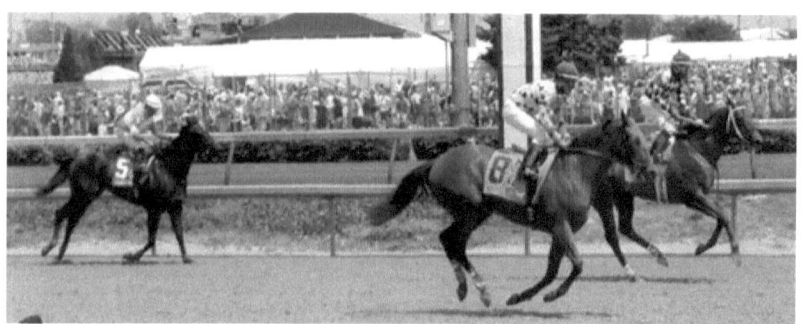

Social Media Note

Did you know there are only four "Commonwealth" states? One of my favorite half marathons came in one of these unique locals. It is my half marathon state #5, charismatic Kentucky! Note that the other commonwealths are Virginia, Pennsylvania, and Massachusetts.

Video Transcript

Bottom line up front, this was one of my very favorite races ... ever! I arrived at the hotel in the evening after driving through Florida, Georgia, Tennessee, and Kentucky. By the way, Tennessee and Kentucky are absolutely beautiful states. I carefully set all of the needed clothes and other things on the small table, so it would be ready in the morning. I looked at the weather which indicated a start temperature of 50 degrees. I pulled out the blue sweatshirt and suddenly found myself hesitating to use it. Two weeks ago, my son wore this over-shirt in the Hollywood half and I knew that if I used it that it wouldn't come back with me. For some reason this bothered me; since it was a piece of our shared history in that great race. In the end, I set it on the table, so I could make the decision in the morning. After everything was in place, I set three different clocks for 5:30am. I woke up just before the alarm trio sounded and preemptively turned them off. As anticipated, the temperature was 50 degrees. After some deliberation I chose my red long-sleeved "Top of Utah" shirt. Then I looked again at the sweatshirt. It was cold. I finally took it with the intention to make the final decision once I got there. After arriving, I got out of the car and pulled on the sweatshirt. The sun wasn't quite up yet as I walked to the starting line. It's always amazing to me how the event becomes more and more real and glorious as you approach the venue. This was no exception. Over the music someone was doing a great job MC'ing and getting everyone excited. He said there would be more than 16,000 people on the track with representation from all fifty states and five countries. This event was HUGE. Just before the start, I took the sweatshirt off, folded it neatly, and set it in a quiet corner hoping to find it after the race. They then bugled "Call to Post"; it is the classic melody by which thoroughbred horses have been called to the post ten minutes prior to race time for well over a century. It is the brief version of the old "Boots and Saddles" tune. The sun was coming up over the buildings as the gun fired and we were off. I noticed the 3:40 marathon pacer 20 feet ahead of me. I was running the half marathon, but both races shared the same track for over 8 miles. I knew that was too fast for me, but I followed him anyway. Sure enough, my first mile was too fast (around 8 minutes), I slowed a bit, but not enough, the next few miles were all under 8:30. I began to feel that I really needed to slow down. It is at this point in many races that I think of my daughter's phrase, "He's coming in hot." For me, this means that you are operating in the "faith zone." Just fast enough to surpass what you have ever done before. I looked at my heart rate. Average of 160, higher than usual. I was feeling like I was willing to lay it on the line, so I left the throttle open. It was at this point that I looked at my watch and saw something that surprised me; I was a mile further than I thought I was! Trust me, that never happens. I was getting tired and I wondered if I could keep up the pace. It was then that we rounded the corner and saw Churchill Downs, the home of the distinguished Kentucky Derby. I don't know what I was expecting but I found myself completely unprepared for the majesty of it all. I forgot about myself for a few minutes as we entered this gigantic and historic venue to run around the inside track. As we exited the stadium, I continued the daunting task of identifying the next person to catch and pass. It is so easy to get lazy in the last miles and just settle in behind someone. I was giving it my all but holding back just enough so I could "come in hot" at the finish line. It was at this point I caught an older gentleman running. His shirt read, "running in memory of my wife". I can't tell you why this affected me so powerfully at the time, perhaps it is because this older gentleman was giving his all in a cause more powerful to him than a cause ever could be. I slowly passed him and kept running hard. To me, my daughter's "running hot" phrase also means "finish it", no matter how hard it is. I was running on empty, but I sped up. I looked at my watch. To my surprise, I had a shot at a PR. My previous PR was a downhill race with a serious grade, so I was surprised I had a shot to beat the time. It's always a gamble on when to start the sprint at the finish line. I turned the corner; the finish line was 100 yards away and there were more spectators than I've ever seen at a race. I ran a few more yards and then flipped the switch to my Tom Cruise sprint. I was now running on "whatever's left". In your mind you think, "ok, prepare for a fast burn, jettison whatever's left in the tank, the finish line is the collapsing point." I probably passed 50 people in that last 75 yards. An audience always appreciates effort, and this was no exception. There was an audible rise in the decibel level as I flew to the finish. A new PR by just under a minute. All these factors contributed to a race I will never forget. There will always be a special place in my heart for this memory. As I slowly walked back to my car, I almost accidentally came again to the quiet corner I had neatly folded and left the blue sweatshirt. It was gone.

https://youtu.be/ICe2rs-1KU0

CO FORT COLLINS TRAIL HALF
The Centennial State

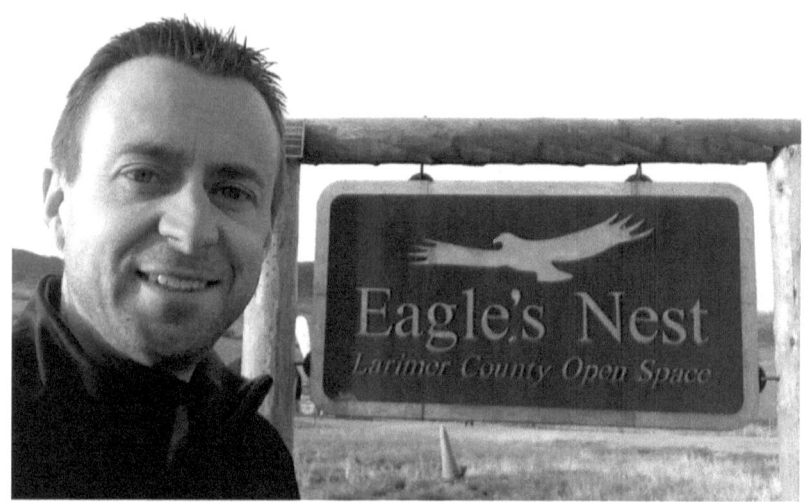

SOCIAL MEDIA NOTE

What do Pikes Peak, Vail, the Broadmoor, the Molly Brown House, and the storied Denver Broncos all have in common? That's right, you'll find them all neatly tucked away in colorful Colorado! And a tip of the hat goes to John Denver and Rocky Mountain High ... Half Marathon state #6 ... check!

VIDEO TRANSCRIPT

State #6 was my fourth half marathon in four states in four weeks. It was also my first of several trail half marathons that I ran. I spent the race-eve night in Denver and got up early to drive the following morning to the Eagle's Nest trail head just northwest of Fort Collins. We were truly out in the sticks. The only building for miles was a Christian church across the street from the starting line. The fact that we were running straight up the mountain right off the bat had me seriously wondering if I had made a grave mistake. After the first few miles, the trail forced us single file which continued for most of the way on this out and back. No arguments from me though, I count myself extremely lucky to escape with my life on this one. Here's to Colorful Colorado, the Eagles Nest, and Rattlesnake Road. Cheers!

https://youtu.be/vPA3IMy5Kcc

TN Viola Valley Half

The Volunteer State

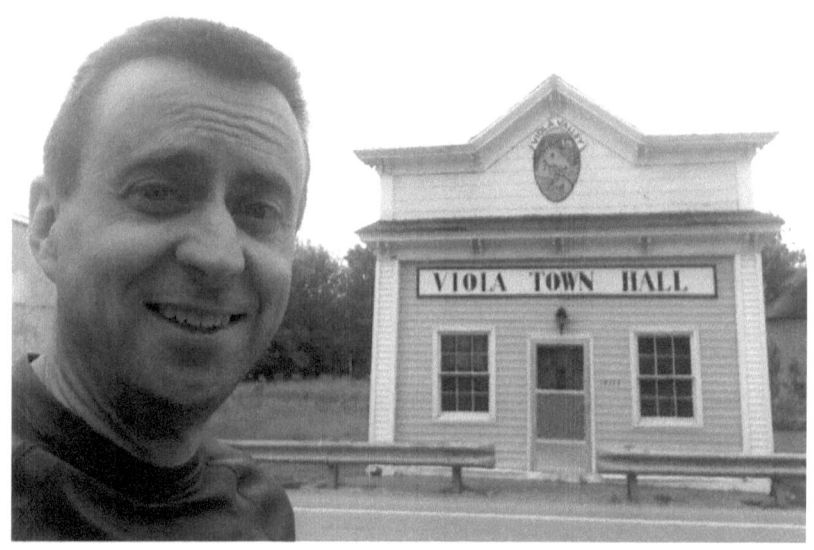

Social Media Note

For #7 I was in the heart of country music land. Home to Nashville's "Grand Ole Opry" and Elvis Presley's Graceland. Also, the home to some of the friendliest people you'll ever meet. I'm blessed to have donated 20,000 steps to the country roads of the great state of Tennessee.

Video Transcript

This race was so much fun. I was so far in the backwoods of Tennessee that it was truly southern accent heaven. I still remember walking up to the town square gazebo, which was about the only building, and pulling out my license for the race packet lady. She looked at it, and then with delight and in the thickest accent ever she said, [Imitated Southern Accent] "You're from Utah? I saw your registration come through. Don't you worry, we have someone from Oregon and someone from Maine." I talked with the registration folks for a bit and walked away just grinning. Later that night I ate at the Cracker Barrel where I happen to be playing Letterpress with my wife across the network. A high-school aged southern speaking waitress walked up to my table where I explained I was playing this word game with my wife back in Utah. She donned a look of dismay and said, [Imitated Southern Accent] "The things they can do now." The next morning, I lined up with the other racers to run through the rolling hills of rural Tennessee. I still remember as I came upon the last mile I sped up to pass someone who quickly decided to make a two-man race of it. We both sped up stride for stride for most of the last mile until, and against my will, I let him pull ahead. I think that last half marathon mile (about 7 minutes) is my fastest final mile I've ever done or ever will do. What a beautiful state and a great experience.

https://youtu.be/zuMgN0vCLOc

ID TETON DAM HALF

The Gem State

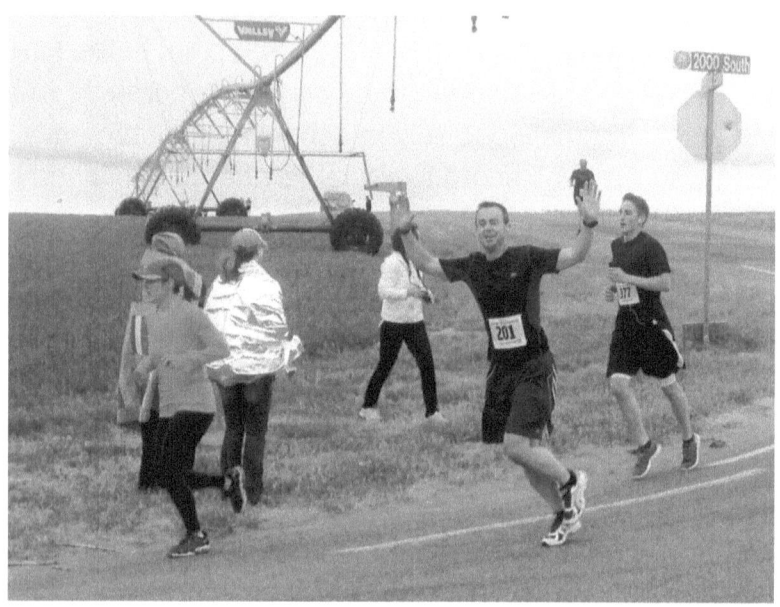

SOCIAL MEDIA NOTE

State #8 half marathon brought me back to the land of my nativity ... and memory lane. Being raised in Idaho, this run will always hold a special place in my heart. Especially because it is associated with the Teton Dam. I was a young lad in south Rexburg when the dam broke, and I was among the many frightened children who listened to the radio as they urged people to get to high ground. I remember my dad moved the food storage from the basement to the main floor and then we left. Luckily, the waters missed our house by 400-500 yards. That was many years ago. This race took me through some of the same areas I was so familiar with as a boy. I was fortunate in this race to have my parents with me. An enjoyable and freezing time was had by all!

VIDEO TRANSCRIPT

Now I know what it must have been like to climb the Tower of Babel. Rexburg's Teton Dam run is aptly named and boasts uphill grades for about the first eight to nine miles with the bulk of the elevation gain starting at mile three or so. They had us running through the dry farms at the apex, and I felt I was running through memory lane as I use to move sprinkler pipe as a boy in these vast fields of grain and potatoes. My nephew Ben also ran this race. I did reasonably well up the ascent, but the climb left my calf muscles oddly and sometimes painfully spasming on the 4-mile descent to the finish line. As a result, my nephew Ben made up some serious ground on me during the final miles of the run. In fact, if there had been 100 more yards he would have beat me but there wasn't, and he didn't. Age luckily won in the end (as it should). My parents, a few sisters, and in-laws were there to see the action. I'm still confused how it can be so cold in the morning in Rexburg in June ... those from Rexburg just smile at that statement and think, "you're lucky it wasn't snowing."

https://youtu.be/iHXb2A-5FAU

MI Grand Island Trail Half
The Wolverine State

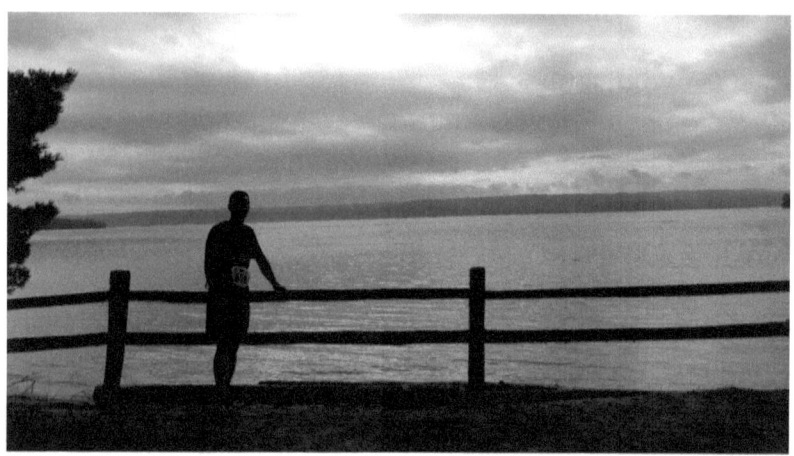

Social Media Note

Ever run around on an island in Lake Superior? I have. My wife was with me for state #9 ... Marvelous Michigan!

Video Transcript

What can I say about Michigan ... this run just might have been my favorite adventure. My wife and I drove up to Lake Superior from Dayton OH. We stopped in Kirtland to see some of the church sites and then headed up to the top of the nation. About five hours north of Detroit you cross the magical place where several of the Great Lakes meet just above Mackinaw. After crossing the bridge to the Upper Peninsula, you start seeing signs for Pasties about every block. We later learned that these pasties are made by placing the uncooked filling, typically meat and vegetables, on one half of a flat short-crust pastry circle, folding the pastry in half to wrap the filling in a semicircle and crimping the curved edge to form a seal before baking. The tradition comes from England, and Michigan's Upper Peninsula is one of the only places in the US where they are sold on every street corner. We took the opportunity to sample these strange entrees near the race start town in Munising. We found them tasty but a bit bland ... still, it's fun to experience the unique foods from different parts of the country. After eating we enjoyed exploring this unique rustic town. In the morning we joined the runners for the short ferry ride from Munising out to Grand Island in Lake Superior. I really can't describe how amazing this was with the sun coming up over the lake and the stunning vistas on the island. That said, no place is pure paradise, and the hummingbird-sized mosquitos were out in force. Luckily, I was able to borrow some repellent, and I wasn't really bothered after that. I was proud of myself for this event because it was a hard trail run and I was fortunate to bring such a strong effort. Here's to Michigan's Upper Peninsula, Lake Superior, and Grand Island. I'll never forget you!

https://youtu.be/Q27oURHWAG4

HI KAUAI HALF
The Aloha State

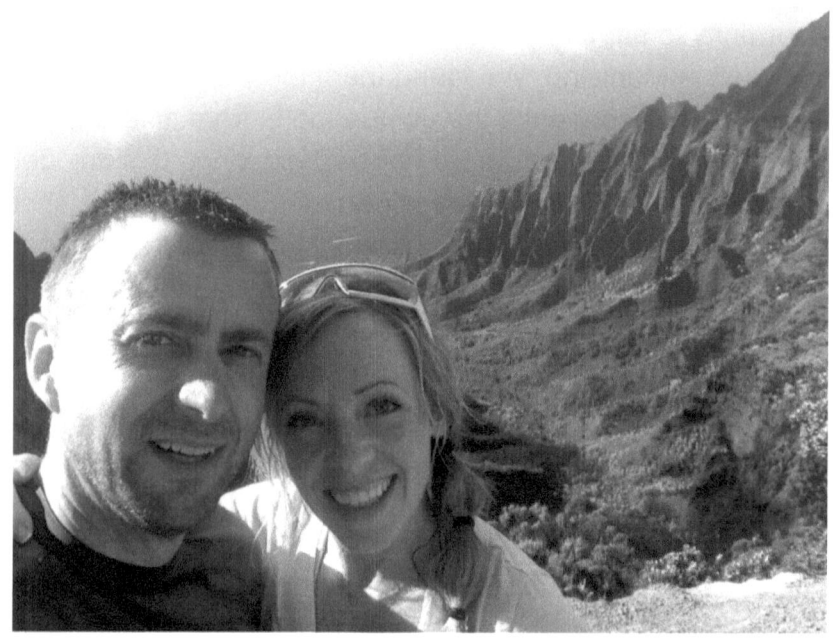

SOCIAL MEDIA NOTE

Hmmm. Let's see ... what was that island state? I remember
my wife and daughter were with me for this one ... the locals
said 'aloha' a lot ... oh yeah, it was the Pacific's grand
Hawaiian islands ;). Here's to that wonderful and warm
tropical paradise of #10 Hawaii's Kauai.

VIDEO TRANSCRIPT

After spending a week on Oahu with our daughter, we drove
to the airport, put her on a plane back to Utah and then we got
on a plan to Kuaui. This was our second trip to Kuaui, but we

adventured like it was our first. We hiked a challenging trail near the end of Waimea Canyon to get great views of the Na Pali Coast, spent a lot of time at the Poipu beaches, swam with sea turtles on the North Shore on Tunnels Beach, swam in Queens Bath, and kayaked and hiked up to Secret Falls. Hawaii was just amazing.

https://youtu.be/W6OZC2OSDCQ

MD Run4Shelter Half
The Old Line State

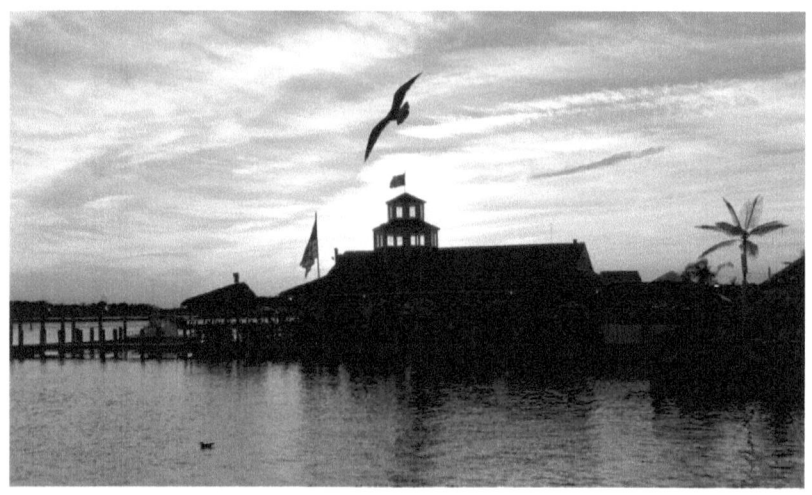

Social Media Note

What state do I spend the most time in aside from Utah and Virginia? Well, that would be #11, Maryland. With the highest median household income in the nation, everything is expensive; no wonder I had to sleep in my car ;).

Video Transcript

This Christian sponsored race was run on Kent Island in Maryland. This was my third of four islands in a row. The first being Michigan's Grand Island, the second Kuaui, this one on Kent Island, and the next (which was on Johns Island, I'll let you look up the state). I slept in a van on this one. It was one of the most miserable nights I've ever spent. I must have felt good though because my time was excellent. Earlier in the week, I did a warmup run at Great Falls, it was beautiful.

[Moments after the race]

Well, we made it all the way to the end. It was pretty crazy out here. It was absolutely beautiful, cloud-covered, perfect conditions for running ... but boy, every time you do it, it's a long, long way. Anyway, I had a lot of fun. I have my medal ... Run 4 Shelter. There are lots of really friendly people out here. Hey, we'll talk to you later.

https://youtu.be/9aqI03RhSs0

SC Lowcountry Trail Half

The Palmetto State

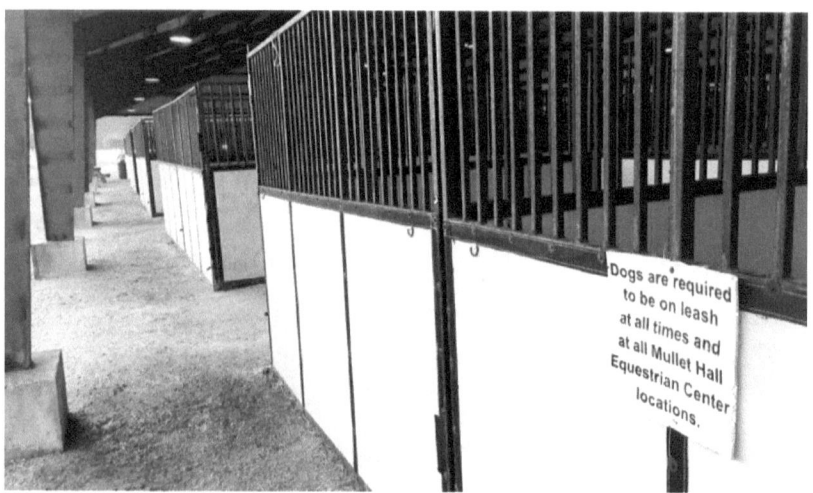

Social Media Note

The Angel Oak, Mullet Hall Equestrian Center, and the Battle of Bloody Bridge are all part of the magic and history of Johns Island. The former two I personally experienced within state #12, delightful South Carolina!

Video Transcript

I drove down from Washington DC one Friday afternoon to run this unique half marathon. I'd never set foot at (let alone on) an equestrian anything before and the Mullet Hall Equestrian Center did not disappoint. The breathtaking fall foliage, moss-draped oaks, and native wildlife provided a beautiful backdrop for this once in a lifetime experience. I arrived a bit early. Ground fog attended the early-morning quiet at this scenic venue.

[Moments before the race]

Good morning. Here we are at the equestrian park in South Carolina. There are mosquitos here and I have no way to fight them. At any rate, it's about an hour and a half before the race. I'm here a little bit early. It's an absolutely beautiful morning. There is mist everywhere hugging the ground. You can't see it right over here but if I turn this way it's beautiful and this phone is not capturing it too great. Anyway, talk to you soon. Hopefully I'll make it through this trail half marathon. See ya. Bye.

[Moments after the race]

I'm alive and kickin'. That was a great race. Third trail run. I thought I'd finally get the two-hour monkey off my back; which means I haven't run over two hours since the first one but I got in just under the two-hour mark. I guess I'm on my way to Charleston airport. Have a good one. Bye.

https://youtu.be/Ii6iM2L-Cmc

IN   MUNCIE MINI

The Hoosier State

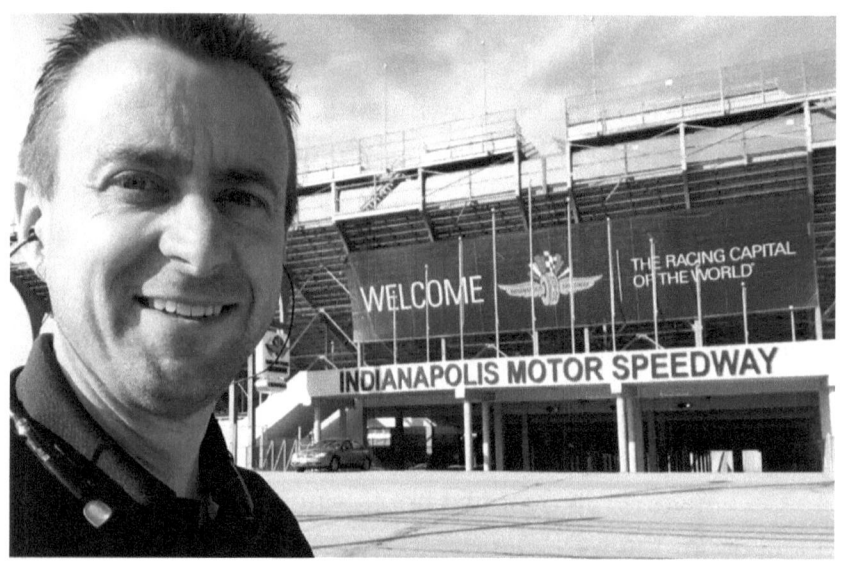

SOCIAL MEDIA NOTE

The mysterious White River, Cardinal Greenways, Minnetrista Cultural Center and Craddock Wetlands ... where else could I be but illustrious Indiana! I drove a long way for the privilege of running in my lucky 13th half marathon state, and it was worth every mile! A tip-of-the-hat goes to the enchanting town of Muncie, I hope I can donate more footfalls to your ideal spot on the Earth sometime down the road.

VIDEO TRANSCRIPT

After walking around and ascending the famous Gateway Arch in St. Louis, I began my sojourn to nearby Indiana. After arriving in Indianapolis, I spent some quality time at the well-known Indianapolis Speedway. They had all kinds of cars in the museum portion (like hundreds) ... they even had a few originals from the first race in 1909. I only spent about an hour at the speedway since it was late when I arrived. After that I made the quick 20-minute drive to Muncie to pick up my number and orient myself to the starting line. When I was satisfied I drove back to my hotel for some sleep. The race the next morning was a beautiful river run that I thoroughly enjoyed.

[Moments after the race]

Hey, we are finishing up in the shadow of Muncie City Hall. It was a great race. We ran along the river almost the whole time. Just fabulous temperature. It was great. I finished in just under 1:52. Just for fun last night we parked in the high school parking lot. So, these are the purple Muncie Central Bearcats and they were just lining up for their football game. So, it was kind of cool. There were a lot of people in the stands and I walked over to find out where to go for what I was doing. I asked them if they were winning and they said, "well we haven't started yet." I said, "well are you favored to win?" And they said, "well, we are playing a team that is ranked #2 in the state. So, it'll be a tough time." So, I checked the score this morning. Muncie did lose 61 to 7. But anyway, it's just been great. It's like a little college town. Here we are at the high school and I'm at the City Hall and the finish line. Have a great day.

https://youtu.be/hz1wGEtWxo8

VA STAR CITY HALF

The Old Dominion

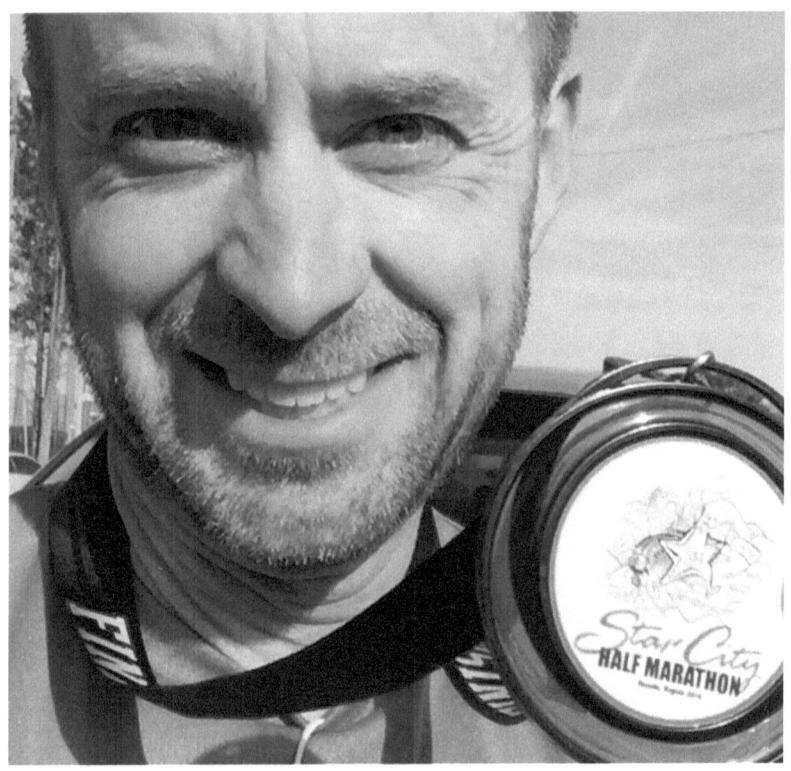

SOCIAL MEDIA NOTE

Ahhh, my home away from home. Sweet #14 Virginia … sigh.
Well, it's about time ;-)

VIDEO TRANSCRIPT

I drove from New Jersey through Pennsylvania and West
Virginia before finally arriving in Roanoke on this cold end-of-
November day. I had falsely assumed that the cold weather

wouldn't be a concern. The morning of the race it was like stepping into icy water itself. Note that I left the second video in the sequence even though I look and act slightly inebriated. Also, lest I receive any hate-mail, let me just make the statement before the videos that I think the people of West Virginia and Virginia are good people. Enjoy!

[Early morning just outside the hotel]

Wow. It's the Commonwealth of Virginia this time, and it is freezing. It is like 27 degrees right now. I am completely unprepared for this cold. I'm going to see if there is a Walmart or something I can go get some stuff, but I am serious, just walking out to the car, my toes are frozen! It is freezing! So, we'll see how this goes, but this is ... I'm not prepared for this. We'll see what happens ... Cheers!

[Moments before the race]

You don't think this is freakin' cold ... grow a brain man. All right, we are about to start. I managed to get a cap and some gloves. It is really, really cold. Okay, about to start, see ya. Bye.

[Moments after the race]

The beginning temperature was 25 degrees. The ending temperature was 30 degrees. Time 1:55. Good run. Cold run. I was going to say, "good people" but I think that the people of West Virginia and Virginia are unique people. Anyway, they are really great. Time to go. See ya. Bye.

https://youtu.be/RqBaUa6lg1o

NY Fred Lebow Central Park Half
The Empire State

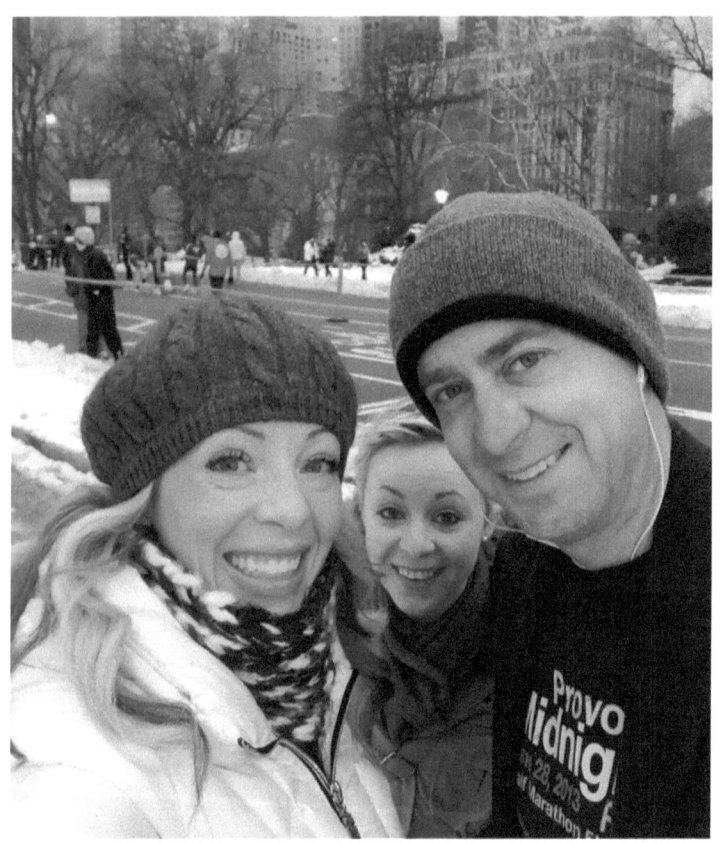

Social Media Note

Only 25 days after New Year's Day blanketed the Big Apple, my wife, daughter and I found ourselves in the city and state everyone wants to visit … #15 New York, New York. Broadway, Ground Zero, Trinity Church, Carlo's famous Bake Shop … and I must mention Juniors where the side order of Mac-and-Cheese combined with your choice of cheesecake never disappoint! To top it off, my awesome brother was able to spend some time with us as well showing us this great city that he gets to call his backyard.

VIDEO TRANSCRIPT

Manhattan, Matilda, the Empire State Building, Ground Zero and Times Square. Where else could we be but New York, New York. My wife, daughter and I boarded a plane to New York where we immediately began seeing the sights. As we approached one of New York's most famous buildings, I thought to myself, "who doesn't race to the top of the Empire State Building with 'An Affair to Remember' playing softly in the back of their minds?" Later in the day, we visited my brother's apartment where he then accompanied us to several sites in and near lower Manhattan including Trinity Church and Ground Zero. In the late evening, we attended the Broadway show, Matilda. It was terrific. They had a man in women's garb play the part of Mrs. Trunchbull which in addition to being hilarious was perfect. The next day we arrived early at Central Park to prepare for and start the race. In hindsight, I can't think of a better place to snag my New York half marathon than Central Park! This was my first race where my daughter was with me, so her feelings were tender as she saw her old man race across the finish line. It just made it that much better! After the race, we drove down to Washington DC by way of New Jersey and Carlos' famous Cake Boss cake shop. I had a red velvet cupcake. On to DC where we saw the sights and called it a trip.

https://youtu.be/UVbIUj4n8E0

WA THE OAT HALF

The Evergreen State

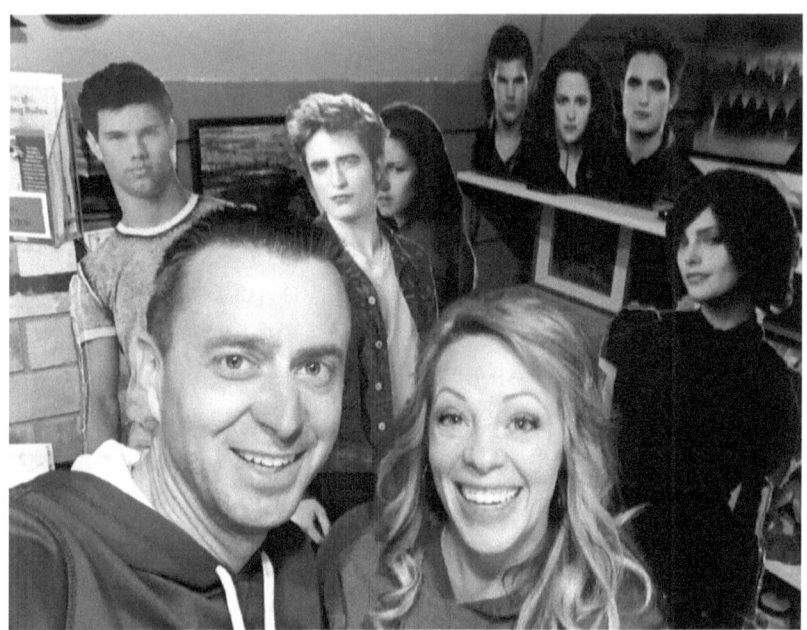

SOCIAL MEDIA NOTE

Okay, Twilight/Vampire fans, this half marathon is for you! Little did I know when I signed up for the infamous OAT run in Port Angeles, that my excursion through half marathon state #16 would be so unique and satisfying. Yup, my wife and I donated several footfalls to Forks and La Push as well. Add that to my totally made-up vampire/human race rules, set in the beautiful Washington Olympic Mountains, and you have a crazy and memorable journey.

VIDEO TRANSCRIPT

After a day or two in Seattle, my wife and I found ourselves up in the Olympic Mountain Range on the Olympic Peninsula of western Washington. This is some of the most beautiful country you will ever see. It is also some of the wettest country you will ever see. In fact, it rained almost constantly as we visited Forks and La Push. To say it was raining was an understatement. When we visited La Push, it was a torrential downpour. Still, I got out of the car to take a picture of the ocean. I was soaked in seconds and the wind almost broke my umbrella. The picture of the Twilight crew is at the Chamber of Commerce in Forks. We quickly learned that Forks is Twilight themed 24/7 and even has a Stephanie Meyer day. The actual run was in Port Angeles. After watching the race videos I've had people ask me if the vampires vs. runners was a real thing. Well, as it turns out, you have a lot of time to think before and during a two-hour run. I made the whole thing up.

[Moments before the race]

All right, here I am in Port Angeles ready to run the half marathon. It looks pretty crazy out here. We're running through the forests here by Port Angeles. You know, in the last couple of days I've spent some time here in Port Angeles and nearby in Forks. I found out from the Indian tribe over there, Jacob and buddies, that evidently the vampires that are running through here during the time we're all here are going to give us a sporting chance. They gave us some paintball guns and I said, "like that's going to do anything." But they said that the vampires are going to give us a sporting chance. So, I've got my gun here and really I just need to keep a human between me and the vampires. I'm just hoping there's less of them then there are of us and then maybe I've got a sporting chance. Anyway, we are about to start in just a few minutes so if I see you on the other side it means I made it. See you later. Bye.

[Moments after the race]

Wow, so that's the OAT run. You know, it seemed weird to me when they just gave us paint-guns at the start with the vampire thing. But, as it turns out, they had safe zones and zones where they could only go so many miles an hour. There was a five mile-per-hour area and a thirty mile-per-hour area. I only had two close encounters. At one of those thirties [thirty mile-per-hour zones] I was going to the five [five mile-per-hour zones] and there were puddles everywhere and I slipped down. You can see them coming at you, because they must go a little slower, and I got up and started going. I was across the five and he just didn't stop. Right before he got me Carlisle zoomed in and caught this guy and then went on. I did pretty good for almost the rest of the way and then I came to another part where I was behind somebody, and it was single file. I was the one in back. All of a sudden, I see this vampire from the tree. He comes zooming in. I duck. He grabs my over-shirt and it comes off. He comes back at me. Jasper hits him from the side. He grabs the shirt back for me and runs up and he gave it back to me. See, here it is. Straight from Jasper. Thank you, sir. All right, anyway it was a good run. About 1:50. Talk to you soon, bye.

https://youtu.be/5choWYfR9ks

NC NEW RIVER HALF
The Tarheel State

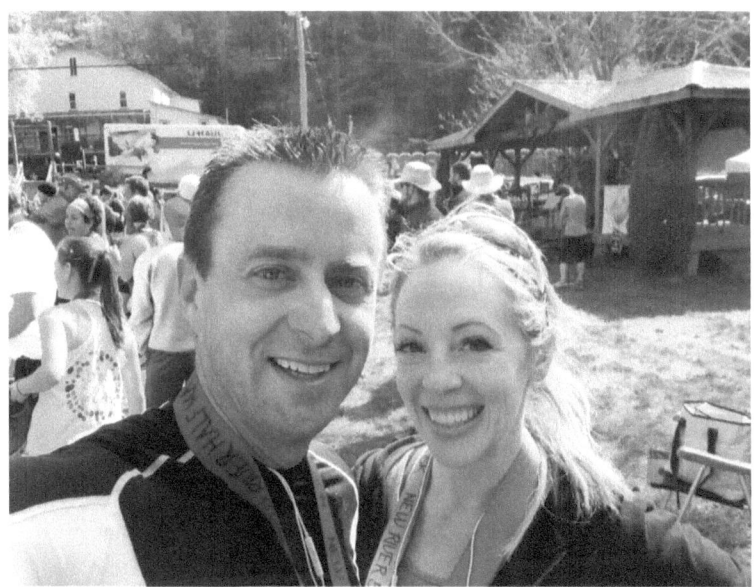

SOCIAL MEDIA NOTE

One day my wife and I found ourselves within the beautiful Blue Ridge Mountain Range in a tiny town with the same name as our oldest son. That's right, half marathon state #17 came in the enchanting town of Todd, North Carolina. We found this little town to be a most charming area, undisturbed from the trouble and cares of the world.

VIDEO TRANSCRIPT

Here we are in Todd, North Carolina. It took us a long time to get here but boy is it beautiful. I'm just going to spin around and show you the great river. They call this the New River.

Yesterday we came up here and it was like going into yesterday up there. So, we went into the Todd Mercantile where they had this metal pressed against the side of the buildings and even on some of the ceilings inside. We paid 30 bucks to go get some pasta that was unremarkable, but it did the job. That's what we're running on. All right. See you after the race.

[Moments after the race]

Wow, quite a race. Here we are at the end. My wife won ... uh. [my wife plays along] "I won!" [Me] My wife ran the 5K and I ran the half. It seemed like it was uphill the whole way. In fact, there were three heart-break hills and believe me they were heart-breaking. It seemed like it was uphill the whole way but how beautiful is this? [Wife] It was awesome. My first race back after a year after my surgery. Slow, but I'm glad I finished it. [Me] So I passed my first marathoners, they started 15 minutes before us, at about mile 4. I learned that there's something you should do if you are bringing up the rear of your race to draw attention from yourself. I noticed that when people where passing them that they were asking them something (this couple that was going slow on the marathon). Finally, when I got to them, I was huffing and puffing past them and they looked over and said, "are you ok, are you ok." I'm like, "Yeah, I'm fine." Well I'm going to have to remember that when I'm in last place and people come by I'm going to just ask them how they are. All right. Have a great one. This has been a great race in North Carolina in the Blue Ridge Mountains. See ya. Bye.

https://youtu.be/2cKUoF2LAUQ

AL Oak Mountain Half
The Heart of Dixie

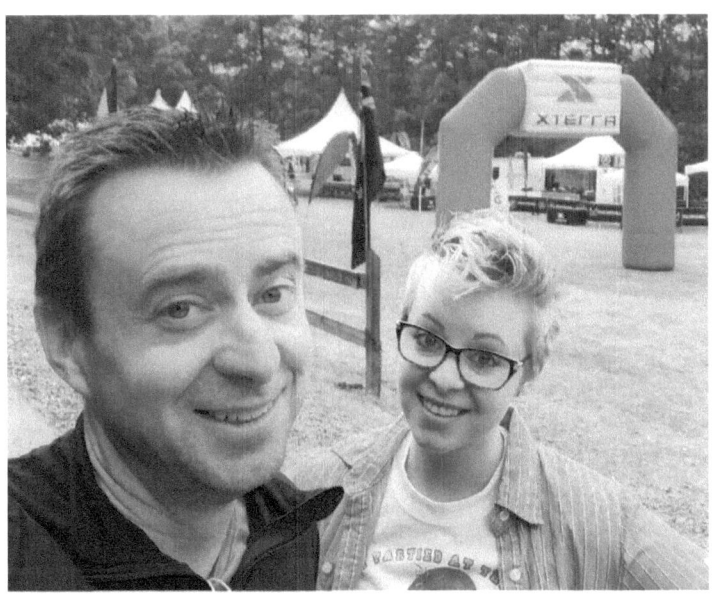

Social Media Note

How appropriate that this week I share the half marathon that helped spark the flame that has become the marriage-fire my daughter and her beau celebrate today. Little did I know when I asked her along on this adventure that there was a secret curiosity working inside her adorable little heart. An innocent curiosity that would only be satisfied after we parted ways in Tampa … when she turned her attention south … toward Naples, FL. Special thanks to our Florida friend for all she has done in supporting us and the happy couple. My wife and I sincerely appreciate it. Even though I lose my charming little daughter to Florida, I am so glad that she is so glad. I'm also blessed that we had this last daddy-daughter opportunity to enjoy a pleasantly rainy #18 Oak Mountain Half Marathon in Alabama before driving down to Tampa, enjoying a delightful seaside dinner, and then a private stroll on the soft ocean sand of the beautiful Gulf Coast at sunset. Dearest daughter, today I tip my glass to you … cheers! I love you.

VIDEO TRANSCRIPT

Well, here we are in Alabama at the Oak Mountain State Park. As you can see we've got in the background the XTERRA finish line and the starting line. And I'm fortunate to have my daughter with me. Is that fun or what! [Daughter] It's so fun! [Me] It is so fun. We are going to do a little sweep around, so you can see how beautiful it is here. [Daughter] It's beautiful. It's wet. [Me] Yes. This might just be the record for the wettest run that I do and hopefully it won't make my shoes too wet. We'll find out at the end if we are alive or not. So, wish me luck, see you at the end. Bye.

[Moments after the race]

Ok, question. Have you ever been schooled by an 8-year-old in the Oak Mountain 20K race? I suspect the answer is "no." But it's also "no" for me. When we started there was this little girl, she's 8-year's old, and she's running in her 19th half marathon. She takes off, I'm running after her. She loses me, and I finally see her for the first time at the halfway mark; and I willed myself past her. I suspect she'll be finishing here any second. Anyway, just under two hours. 1:59:53. It was an up and down course with plenty of chances to sprain your ankle … which I almost did. All right. Anyway, it looks like Alabama is in the books! Talk to you later. Bye!

https://youtu.be/-DVNtvKA4vw

MA Newburyport River Run

The Bay State

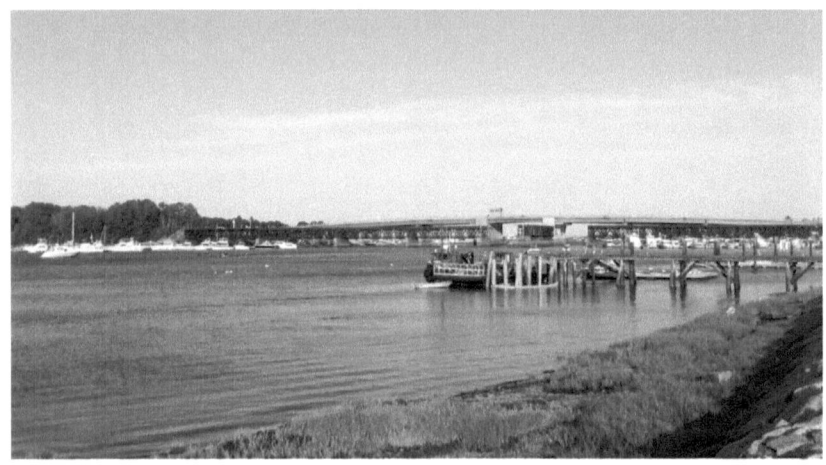

Social Media Note

Less than 60 minutes north of grand ol' Boston lies Newburyport. A historic coastal town that was home to former president John Quincy Adams and claims actors, authors, abolitionists, former Senators, polar explorers and even a signer of the Declaration of Independence among its residents at one time or another during the past four centuries. Also famous for its coastal marshes and its riverfront streets, the town of roughly 20,000 is also the place where the first "Tea Party" rebellion against the British tea tax took place. Here's to half marathon state #19 … Massachusetts!

Video Transcript

Good morning. It's just before the race and a balmy 66 degrees. It feels great out here. This just might be the warmest start I've ever had. Certainly, the warmest I've had in a long time. I'm just in the T-shirt and shorts. I'm in Newburyport Massachusetts which is a small coastal city in Essex County Massachusetts. You can see that I'm here at the harbor where they are parking some of the local boats. The starting line is behind me over there somewhere. I'm going to go and check it out right now. It's going to be a great run. It really feels great. The only bad thing, right, is on Thursday I couldn't even walk on my ankle so it's just a couple of days later and we'll see how it goes. Talk to you soon.

[Moments after the race]

I made it. Wow, I must be just a little bit sick because that was hard. For the last several miles I was fighting a Charley Horse in my right calf. 1:59:55. I'm telling you, I'm flirting with the two-hour mark in every race it seems like now. It was fun. At the outset, you know, for the first couple of miles I tried to answer the prayer that was written on the back of some lady with a ponytail flipping back and forth. The back of her shirt read, "Please let there be someone behind me to read this." I thought that was great, so I was able to fulfill that prayer for her for a few miles and then she pulled away. At any rate, what a great race. If you are feeling good this would be the perfect place to race. It's overcast and about 70 degrees. Humid. You have the sea air coming in hitting you in the face. Just great. All right. Talk to you later. Bye.

https://youtu.be/iWGM5J746_4

MT West Yellowstone Half
The Treasure State

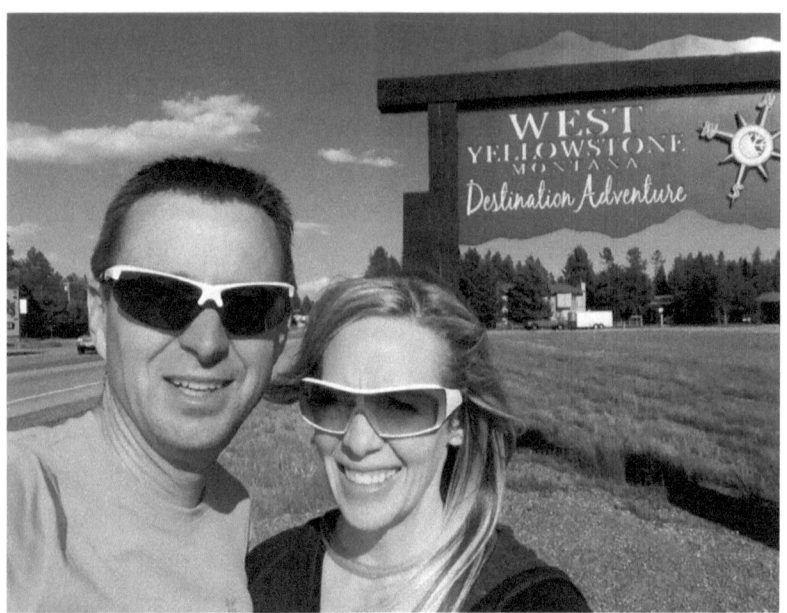

Social Media Note

My wife and I zipped up to the KOA just west of West Yellowstone for this race. Who of us older northern Utahans and southeast Idahoans haven't spent at least one night in this enchanting little mountain town. Whether catching a show at the famous Playmill Playhouse, grabbing ice cream at one of the unique corner stores, or just walking through the charming lodgey-style shops that line the mountain streets. What a pleasure to have experienced half marathon state #20 in the great state of Montana.

Video Transcript

So here we are in West Yellowstone Montana. So, this is state number twenty for half marathons! I'm excited. Today has been great. We had my son's birthday today. We celebrated it a couple of days ago, but we had a great morning with him. On the way up, it was like traveling down memory lane. We passed Fall River, Mesa Falls and Henry's Lake. Now we are at a KOA campground just outside of West Yellowstone. Tomorrow morning at about 6:30 we will start our sojourn into town to the starting line. It's a trail. It said to prepare for tall grass and mud. So that's what I'm going to do. I'm lucky to have my wife with me. She's the one holding the camera. So, we'll see you at the end of the race. Bye.

[Moments before the race]

Wow, here we are at the starting line early in the morning here at West Yellowstone Montana. I don't know if you can see all the people that are here but there are just so many more people here than I ever thought could be here. Now I'm looking at the start line over here and there are so many people. Just a lot of people. Anyway, it should be fun and hopefully [jokingly] there will be enough for all the bears. See ya.

[Moments after the race]

That was a great race. It was uphill. It's nice when you get to the end and you talk to folks who ran the Teton half last week and they say, "that was nothing like this one ... in fact that one was 15 minutes faster." So, it makes me feel good because this one was hard. We went essentially straight up right in the center and then just a steady uphill to the end and I don't know who thinks that's ok; because that's not ok. Anyway, the thing that slows you down the most [jokingly] is just the banging the sticks together to keep the mountain lions and bears away.

That's what really slows you down. Anyway, awesome medal. We'll take a closer picture of it when we make the video. I count myself lucky to be able to be in a place like this and to run. It was really hard, but I did well. 1:58 on a course like this is awesome. So we'll see you on the next one. See ya.

https://youtu.be/-WE8QDa0LBI

NH NH-VT Covered Bridge Half

The Granite State

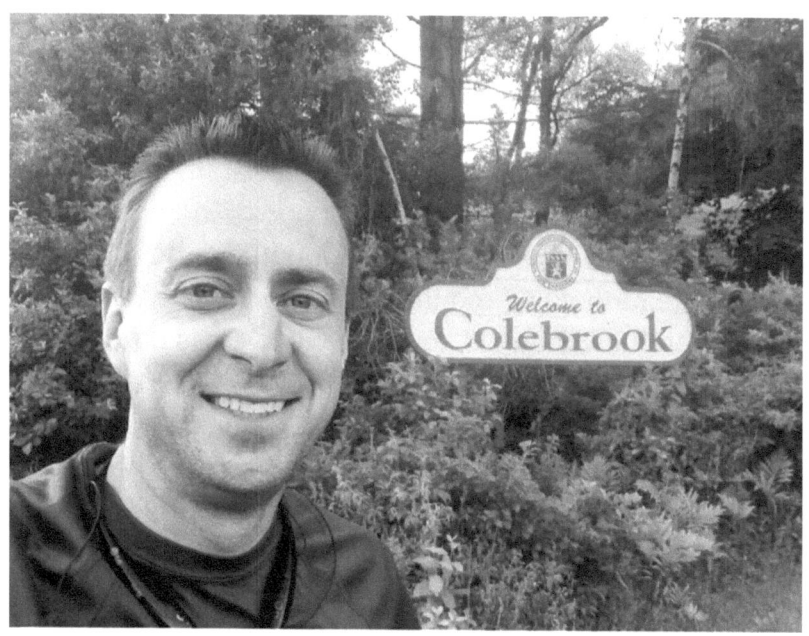

Social Media Note

Situated in the Great North Woods Region, it is bounded on the west by the Connecticut River and home to Beaver Brook Falls Natural Area. The main village of the town is known as Colebrook, and that's where my half marathon state #21 adventure began ... in the charming northern woods of New Hampshire.

Video Transcript

Well, good morning. I'm here before most of the runners. It's kind of interesting how every race is different. This is the latest start I've ever had. So about 10:30am is when they'll start it. Which is late for me this time and it matters because this is the first time I have two in a row. So, I've got a race tomorrow and I need as much time for my legs to recover as possible; but we're just going to worry about today right now. I don't know where I find these races, but they are up in the mountains and just so beautiful. In fact, let's just spin around right here. I wish you could hear all the birds chirping; it's great. In fact, on the way up it's almost like I'm in a magical book. The different places I pass ... like there was Twin Mountains, Stratford Hollow, White Mountain, and the Great Northern Wood. I might be there now, I don't know. Anyway, this is cool. We'll spend some time running in Vermont as well, but the start and end line are in New Hampshire, so New Hampshire gets this one. I'll be back to Vermont another day. Anyway, the race starts in about an hour and a half. I'm wearing my Teton Dam shirt. So, this is my Idaho shirt here in New Hampshire. We'll see how I do. Hopefully it won't be a bad run. It's nice and cool; about 70 degrees. It's about 1000 feet elevation, about the same as the population here in Colebrook. Talk to you after. See you. Bye.

[Moments after the race]

Wow, what a terrific race! I just about haven't been on something so beautiful. It's hard for me to get used to these rolling hills. Wow, but just wildflowers everywhere. We crossed over into Vermont just a quarter mile into the race. Then about 8 miles were run in Vermont. So, I put more footsteps in Vermont than New Hampshire, but the starting and ending line is in New Hampshire. So, it just does my heart good to know that one day I'm going to be back in Vermont and enjoy the scenery again. What a great race. On to the next one. It's about a four-hour drive. I need to go and see if I can get my legs to recover as much as possible because the next race is in about 17 hours. Have a good one. I sure enjoyed New Hampshire. What a great state. Bye.

https://youtu.be/ZSIPwrlGP-A

ME Black Bear Half

The Pine Tree State

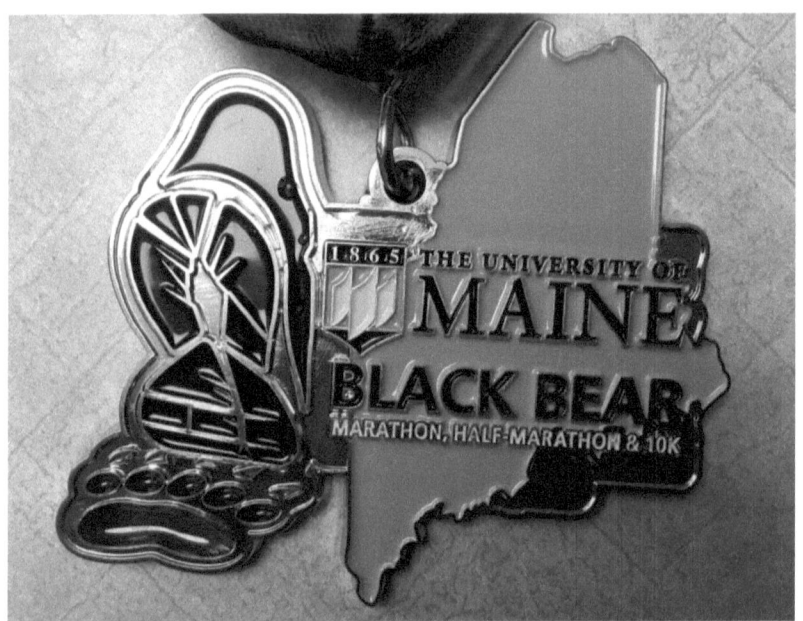

Social Media Note

This was the first time I had ever done two half marathons in two days (this was the second of the two). As a result, I got a little emotional at the end of this one. It was a roller coaster ride of a weekend. This beautiful state is known for its scenery— it's jagged, mostly rocky coastline, low, rolling mountains, heavily forested interior, and picturesque waterways. What's the state with the northernmost Atlantic coastline? You guessed it … Maine!

Video Transcript

I apologize for the wind at the start of the video. It fades after about 15 seconds. I got a little emotional after this race. I had just run in New Hampshire 18 hours earlier and had been really been worried that I wouldn't be able to finish well in this race. In the end this run was extremely taxing and in a torrential downpour the whole time. Despite a constant effort to increase the pace, I had resigned myself that this would be my first race over two hours. I even found myself thinking, "It's ok, it's pouring rain, you ran 18 hours ago, and then you spent all day sitting in a car." Then, when I rounded the corner in the stadium and saw the master clock tick to 1 hour 59 minutes, a smile crawled across my face bigger than you could possibly imagine, I sprinted to the finish and threw my arms in the air. Then, I just broke down. I tried to keep it out of the video, but it didn't work. Thanks for sharing this private moment with me.

[The day before the race]

At any rate, I'm looking forward to tomorrow. My legs are a little bit tired from this morning. We'll see how I do. I don't want to walk. The race director in here said, "Hey I saw your registration. You're clear from Utah." She said, "Don't you worry, you just walk you'll be just fine." Well, I don't want to walk. We men can run our races. Anyway, it's supposed to be bad weather tomorrow. Rainy ... 70 degrees and rainy so maybe that won't be so bad. The good part, right, is that perhaps my stuff will get wet tomorrow and not this morning. Anyway, I'll talk to you again tomorrow. Have a good one. See ya. Bye ... bye!

[Moments before the race]

The race is about to start and everybody is in their cars. I thought the wettest race would be in Alabama. It ended up not raining there. So far, I think the wettest race has been

Massachusetts. It rained for about 20 minutes. Evidently it is forecast to rain hard, 100% chance the entire race. It's downpouring now and I'm going to be one wet boy. I'm going to see how it is to run two in a row. My calf muscles were spasming, waking me up at two or three in the morning. They feel ok right now. So, we'll see how it goes. See you at the end. Bye.

[Moments after the race]

Wow, that was awesome. Nothing really makes you feel so alive. It was a very wet race. It down-poured the entire time. As you know, I ran a half marathon yesterday. I was super worried about it. It was so hard, and I slowed down. I just can't tell you what happened. I didn't have my watch with me. The one that told me the time. I knew I was running slower. As I ran into this stadium and saw the clock ... and it clicked over to 1:59 ... I can't even tell you what went through my head. Anyway, I made it in under two hours. Great race. On to the airport. It's been a great visit here in Bangor, Maine. Talk to you later. See ya.

https://youtu.be/QvbQw7ZE83A

WI   LUNA-TIC HOUND DOG HALF
The Badger State

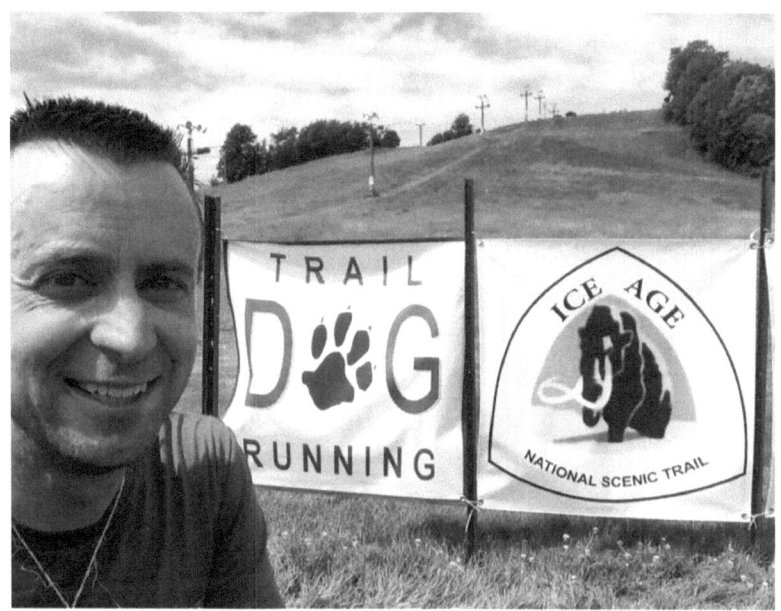

SOCIAL MEDIA NOTE

I didn't learn my lesson in New Hampshire and Maine (never schedule two races in two days). Oh well, it's worth it. In any case, I loved spending 24 hours in this fantastic mid-western state with coastlines on 2 Great Lakes, Michigan and Superior, and an interior of forests and farms. What a pleasure to run in the backcountry of #23 Wisconsin!

VIDEO TRANSCRIPT

All right, I'm not going to get another chance to do this. Here we are in Wisconsin. We are about 30 miles west and 1000 vertical feet from the shores of Lake Michigan. It's hot. I swear

I find every kind of weather to run these things in. It's 72 degrees, and within about an hour it'll be 80 degrees. By some mercy I've got a thunderstorm here; probably for at least half the race, we'll have this thunderstorm going on here. You'll see that I'm at a ski area. This is a key indicator that I'm in the wrong place. So, this was the closest race; there are three half marathons here in Wisconsin, and this was the closest one by several hours. So, I selected this race even though it looks like it's the hardest. It looks like, from the elevation map, it'll be the toughest race I've ever done. Plus, it's got some technical sections that this rain will make slippery and muddy to get through. Anyway, here I am in the middle of the summer in the thunderstorm in the heat at a ski area. This is Sunburst ski area which is really close to West Bend, Wisconsin. Anyway, we'll see how I do. I'll see you at the end.

[Moments after the race]

Well here I am at the end. Wow, that was certainly crazy. I finally did go over two hours, but I am not ashamed at all. This is the hardest race I have ever done. Even harder than Michigan or Washington. It was just hard. Very satisfying though. I guess the next time I'll just have to know that if a race is called Luna-tic Hound Dog Half Marathon and it starts at a ski resort, it's 80 degrees and super muddy ... you know ... choose a different race. This race was fun. At the start there was some thunderstorm activity so they waited to start and so I got the best of both worlds. I got sun, 80 degrees, a hundred billion percent humidity, and the mud. It was like running on marbles. Anyway, I've got to get down to Illinois to get my number for tomorrow. I'm just so glad that I chose this one for Wisconsin. It's just exactly how I'd like to remember it and this will probably be the only time I make it back here to

Wisconsin. Anyway, to the people of Wisconsin, thanks for a great race. I'll see you later. Bye.

https://youtu.be/VFMpZ7hpS2Y

IL   Chicago Rock 'n' Roll Half

The Prairie State

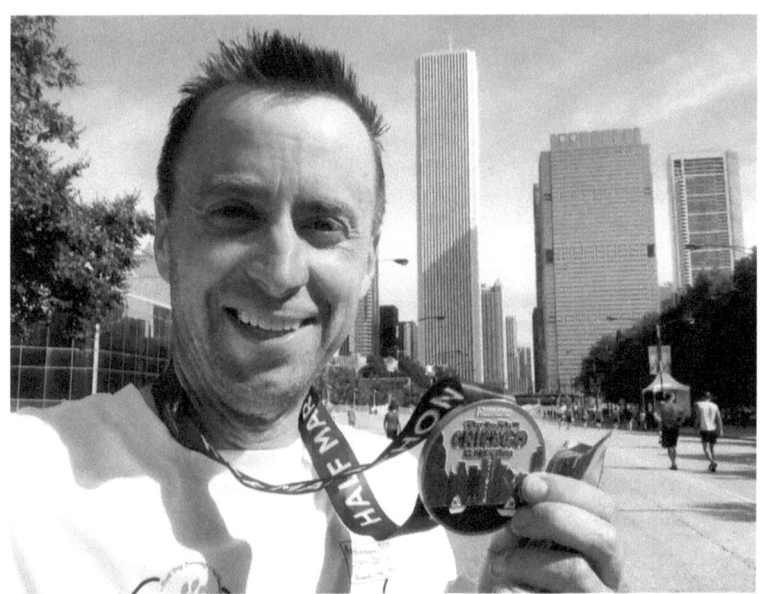

Social Media Note

The day after Wisconsin I find myself smack-dab in the Land of Lincoln. At the starting line in Chicago, I found myself thinking of the Kirk phrase in Star Trek IV, "You're not exactly catching us at our best." Spock chased the comment with, "That much is certain." Despite the cards stacked against me on this one, I loved #24 Illinois!

VIDEO TRANSCRIPT

It was bound to happen sometime. I found myself feeling sick before this race. I had spent my all in a very hot and humid trail race the day before in Wisconsin; and then only got an hour and a half of sleep since I had to start into Chicago at 4am to make it to my parking spot by the required 5:30am. My stomach was upset, and my hands were visibly shaking. It was so hot and humid before the race that I thought I might pass out before the gun even went off. I can truly say it is the first time I've ever really contemplated pulling out of a race. I tried hard to hide it in the video. I even recorded the first part twice because I was shaking so bad; and I wanted it to be a happy moment. It was harder to hide how I felt at the end of the race, but I did a good job. I'm sure I was within minutes of collapsing at the end. It really was all I could do to keep jogging through the heat and humidity.

[Moments before the race]

I don't know how you don't get excited for an event like this. You know, when I found it on the internet I thought, "I want to run here." I love Chicago. I used to come here a lot for work and I haven't been here for a long time. I'm coming here from Wisconsin. I ran in Wisconsin yesterday. It was hot. In fact, someone told me there that yesterday and today are going to be the hottest days in two years. It's hot right now. I only got an hour and a half of sleep, so we'll see how long I can go. I'd like to do well, but you take what you can get ... and what I can get today is a half marathon in Chicago on the shores of Lake Michigan. What more could you want! Anyway, I'll talk to you at the end. I'm excited. See ya. Bye.

[Moments after the race]

Well, I made it through. This is one I'll remember not necessarily because it was super fun but because it was super hard. I have never seen so many people laying on the side of the road. Just laying down with people working on them. Since Goblin Valley I just haven't seen that. I think I ran the end of this race about as dehydrated as I've ever been in my life but that's just how it goes. I have loved being here in Chicago. What a great race. A great venue with Lake Michigan just over yonder. I'll talk to you soon. Have a good one. Bye.

https://youtu.be/RNWWoJ2RWOI

AK Santa Claus Half

The Last Frontier

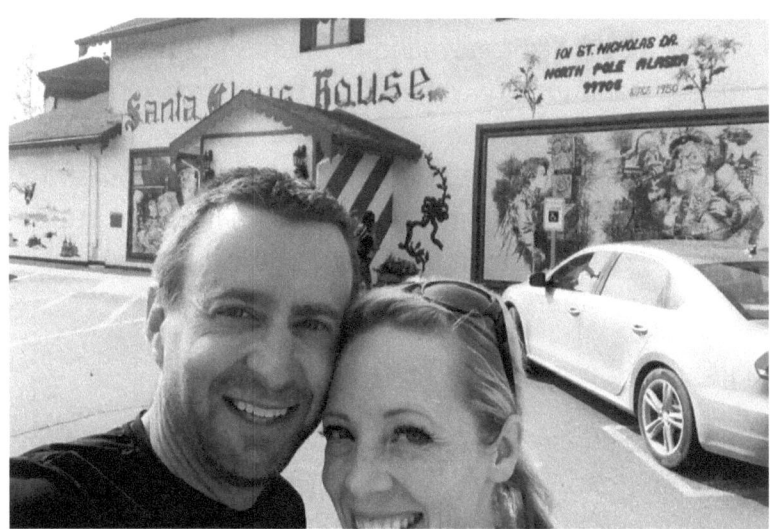

Social Media Note

Which US state has the motto, "The Last Frontier"? Well, here's a hint. It's a vast state. Other notable attributes are that it's breathtakingly beautiful, often cold, and my awesome sister lives there. What a privilege to have Alaska as my half marathon state #25. To top it off, the race was run in North Pole (near Fairbanks) where it is always Christmas-time. It was a perfectly pleasant experience to spend a lazy northern-style week (except for the race), with my wife, sister and her husband.

Video Transcript

Here we are in North Pole Alaska! That's right, that's just 1.3 degrees from the Arctic Circle. No snow today but you'll see it here soon. We are about to line up for the Santa Claus half marathon. I've got the Christmas music all cued up. Excited to go. This will be state #25. I'm so excited! We are about to start and then right afterwards we will tell you how I did. Hopefully it'll be ok. You know it's really kind of interesting here. It's cold for the amount of humidity. When I got up this morning it was 90% humidity and 47 degrees. That's strange. By the start of the race it should be down to about 80% humidity and about 57 degrees. Still, hopefully my muscles will do ok. I'm super excited for this one; to run in the most northern place I will ever run. We will see you at the end.

[Moments after the race]

Ok, who gets to chase Santa Clause on the roads, in the forests, on the trails, on the levees, in North Pole Alaska! Well, it's me! So, I get Christmas in August and I just want you to know that was exactly what I thought Alaska should be like. It was just a complete privilege to run that race. I absolutely loved it! The other great thing about it is it's #25. So now I'm officially half way done and what a great place to do it in Alaska. I love Alaska. See ya.

https://youtu.be/SGWnNjMLO8c

GA Tortoise and the Hare Half

The Peach State

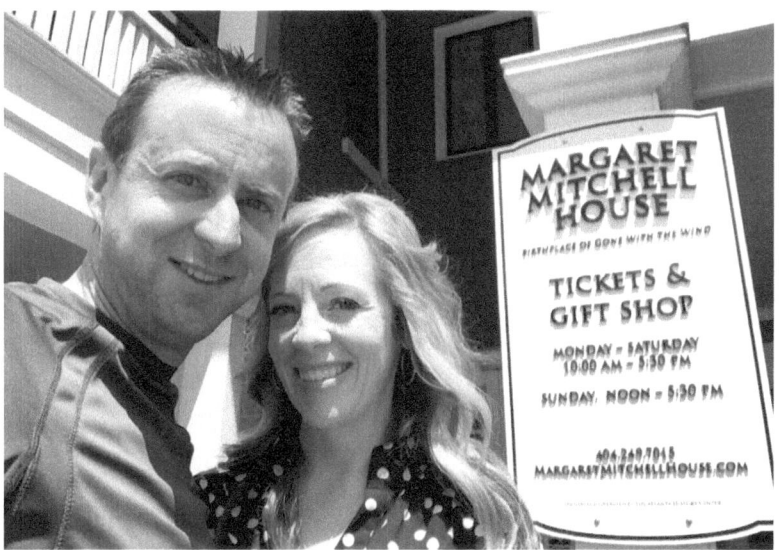

Social Media Note

I can't believe it! I'm starting the last half of my 50-state journey. It feels like getting to the halfway point in a race … the rest will go too fast. That said, I've loved the opportunity to bask in so many great experiences. I truly plan to live in the moment of each state-run and not "look past" it to the next. What a wonderful life … and what a perfect way to start the second 25 than my wife and me spending a few days with our daughter before setting our sights on #26, Georgia … with echoes of Margaret Mitchell's Gone with the Wind in the air.

Video Transcript

I bet from looking around right here that you can't tell that we are in the great state of Georgia. This is green. It's beautiful this morning. I get to run through the foothills of the Blue Ridge Mountains. I'm blessed to have my wife here by my side. It's been fun to have her here. It's kind of scary because it's going to be a high-humidity high-temperature affair, but right now it feels pretty good. We've had a great morning so far. Let's just spin around quick so you can see how great this is. We are where, Wikipedia says, is the heart of the Cherokee Nation, or what used to be the heart of the Cherokee Nation. Anyway, just beautiful today. We are at Cherokee High School. This is the entrance to many of the trails that go into the Blue Ridge Mountains. We just did get a brief from some folks here that said it's easy to get lost. So ... if I'm not back ... [Wife] You'll be back. [Me] All right well we'll see you at the end.

[Moments after the race]

Wow. A little over two hours. It was just absolutely beautiful. There were a lot of little creeks to pass. No one told me it was Sherwood forest back there. There were two trees so covered in a spider web it looked like a giant spider would just come out and eat you! I'll tell you what; I've ran over thirty of these (not states, but like all together) and I have never fallen. I went down twice on this one. Twice ... and I almost tripped once more. So, I've never fallen before but I fell twice. Once at the three-mile mark and once at the ten-mile mark. It was just so slippery but just beautiful. Even though it was really hot and humid your in the trees and so ... you know ... it's a very respectable run, but you can do it! So, I'm just so thrilled that we were here to do Georgia. What a fitting start for second half of my 25 ... this is number 26. Anyway, so we're excited.

Hopefully we'll make it to the airport. It's been fun. We'll see you later.

https://youtu.be/PUjmGvSF458

MN Circle the Lake Half
The North Star State

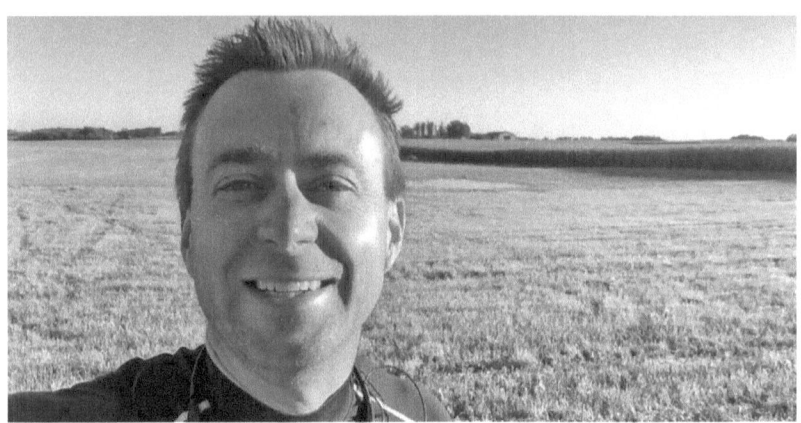

Social Media Note

"Who can turn the world on with her smile? Who can take a nothing day, and suddenly make it all seem worthwhile?" We older folks know that can only be Mary Tyler Moore and WJM-TV in Minneapolis/St. Paul. Minneapolis also happens to be only an hour drive from my 27th state-run in Faribault, Minnesota. What a great opportunity to run around a beautiful lake in the southern part Minnesota. I even ran on the part of the get-away trail of Jesse James' Northfield heist. With only 23 states to go, it looks like "I'm gonna make it after all."

VIDEO TRANSCRIPT

Well, welcome to Minnesota. It just rolls off your tongue ... sounds refreshing. Kind of like a small drink. Anyway, I drove over 700 miles yesterday to be here. I went through five states. Ohio, Indiana, Illinois, Wisconsin and Minnesota. I'm excited about this one. We get to run around a lake called Circle Lake and it's not that little puddle that you see behind me. It's the other direction but you must run to it so I'm not going to get a picture of that right now. I'll tell you that part of the reason that this was interesting is because right up the street a couple of miles is First National Bank. Almost 139 years ago today Jesse James went up there with his gang and robbed that bank. He ran this direction and I'm going to be running on part of the trail that he escaped on. He robbed the bank right up there in Northfield. I'm excited to get started. I'm about a half a mile away from the start line. That's where they had us park, so I need to get over there. I'll talk to you at the end. This is just beautiful as you can tell. Rolling hills, trees, you only get this up here in the north. It's just beautiful. Kind of chilly, 45 degrees. Excited. See you at the end. Bye.

[Moments after the race]

Wow, that was a terrific race. If I could get up every Saturday morning and run that one ... wow! Minnesota, perfect weather, sun is out, 55 degrees, a lot of hills but just a beautiful place. There's something about these northern border-states that just makes me feel at home. Minnesota is no exception. Anyway, thanks for a great race. Off to the airport. I sure have enjoyed it. See ya. Bye.

https://youtu.be/pFb4pm8Ac_s

CT HARTFORD HALF

The Constitution State

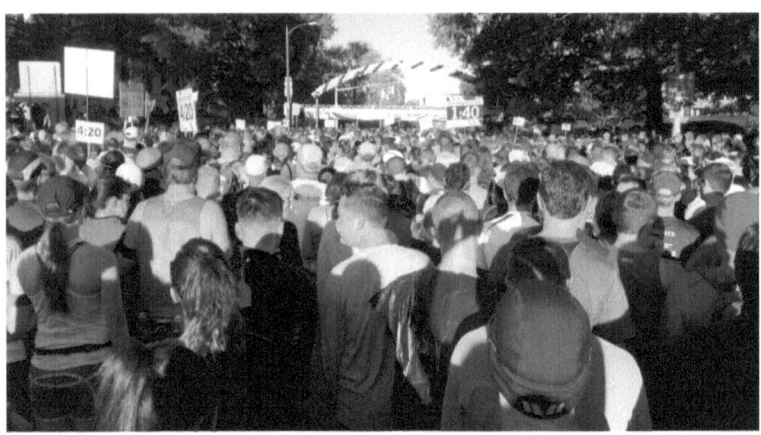

SOCIAL MEDIA NOTE

Here's to the state that published the very first phone book (with only 50 names) … as an aside, about fifteen years ago I spent some quality time at Waterbury in an area we affectionately called Johnny Cake. I remember being continually amazed at how "perfect" the scenery was. I would think, "This scene could be in a Norman Rockwell painting." Then I would look another direction and think it again. It was simply marvelous. Cheers to my #28 state-run in scenic Connecticut!

VIDEO TRANSCRIPT

Well, welcome to the great state of Connecticut. I don't know if you can see the capital right behind me, but we are getting started here at Bushnell Park. We are going to run through the city of Hartford. This is the insurance capital of the world. In fact, I have insurance here. Pretty exciting stuff. Another thing that's kind of interesting is that Mark Twain had a residence here at Hartford for 17 years and, I believe, he wrote parts or all of Tom Sawyer and Huckleberry Finn right here in Hartford. So how fitting a century and a half later that I'm going to be running around in the same place where Tom Sawyer and Huckleberry Finn ran around in the head of Mark Twain. It's a little bit cold this October morning, but I'm super excited. I must go over to the start line and find my spot. This is as big as the Hollywood Half ... about 16,000 participants. So, it should be a really fun time. I look forward to talking to you at the end. See ya. Bye.

[Moments after the race]

Well, here we are, full circle. You know these races are never too bad if you just do one, but I've got another one tomorrow. I've got an injury on my foot, and it doesn't feel too good. It bothered me the last three miles. We'll see if we can get her fixed up for tomorrow, but I just love running in places like this. At mile four or so there's this old guy, must have been 75, he hobbles past me, and he's got like this pumpkin beanie on with argyle socks and shorts. That is so cool! I think that's great. I also like looking at what's written on the shirts. Some are true to life; a good lesson no matter where you are. One said, "pain is temporary but finishing lasts forever." So, in everything you do ... finish it ... finish it well. Anyway, who doesn't want to escape to Connecticut? I mean look at this. This is fantastic! As I'm running on the course, it's fall, and the leaves are slowly falling from the trees onto the roads ... just lined with these beautiful trees. Love Connecticut. On we go to the next one but what a great state! Talk to you later. Bye.

https://youtu.be/jisrzxYI-tc

NJ SHADES OF DEATH HALF
The Garden State

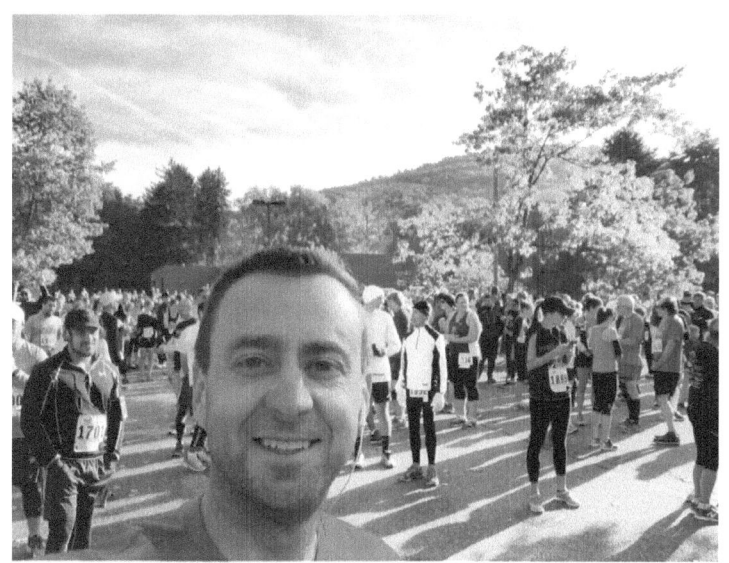

SOCIAL MEDIA NOTE

Ever heard of "Shades of Death Road"? Either had I until I signed up for my Halloween run in rural Allamuchy. Also home to Asbury Park, Wildwood, Atlantic City, Seaside Heights, and Cape May; my 29th state half marathon run in The Garden State of New Jersey was one of the most beautiful (and scary) ever!

VIDEO TRANSCRIPT

Welcome to my Halloween run! It's early in the morning in October in New Jersey at a place called Shades of Death Road. I was going to tell you what I read on the internet about this place, but it is too bad and too scary. So, you'll just have to look it up yourself ("Shades of Death New Jersey Legends"). I'm glad it's an October MORNING because this place is a little spooky. This is a great place to have my Halloween run even though I am running on a hurt foot from yesterday. This is the third time I've done two in a row. The first time I did ok, the second time was kind of a crash-and-burn ... we'll see what it is this time. This time I'm injured but I'm so excited to be in New Jersey's Shades of Death Half Marathon. The shirt is terrific! I'll have to put a picture of that on the little movie that I make. Anyway, I will see you at the end but this should be fantastic. Wildcat swamps, strange happenings, and some pretty bad things have happened around here. Anyway, I'll talk to you at the end. See ya. Bye.

[Moments after the race]

No crash-and-burn today! Wow, I got in behind somebody, and with all my might I tried to follow them no matter what and I *may* have gotten a PR. I think it was 1:48:49 or something. That is really close to my Kentucky PR. I'm just scared that I missed it by a couple of seconds. Who knew that the day after I ran in another state I would come here to New Jersey and run through this beautiful area. What was spooky in the dark is just a visual pleasure in the day. I mean this is just beautiful! I need to go see if I got a PR. I'll be sad if I missed it by a couple of seconds. Anyway, have a good one. What a great run! I just pushed myself hard, and it paid off. I'll see you later. I loved New Jersey. See ya. Bye.

[Editor's note: I missed a PR by only 10 seconds]

https://youtu.be/qRGcuK__Mu0

PA Runners World Half

The Keystone State

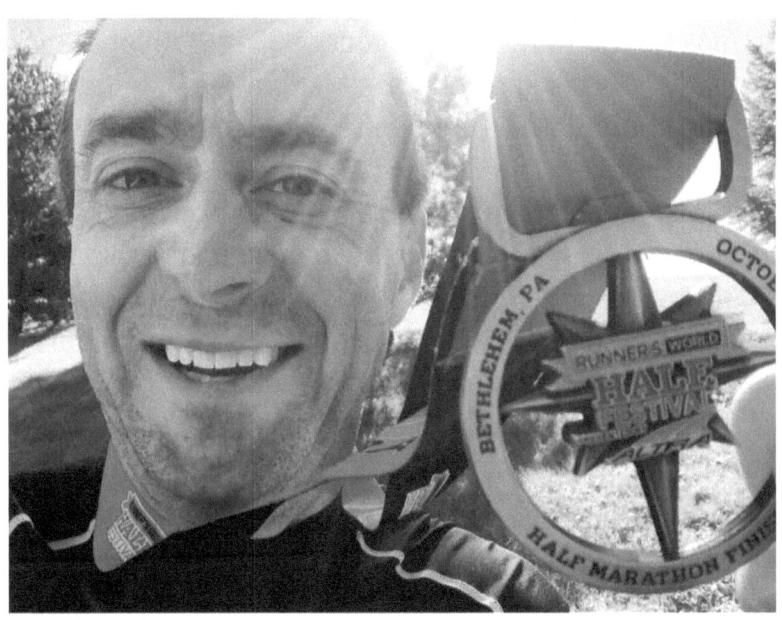

Social Media Note

If I had to choose my most emotionally charged race videos (so far), it would be Maine and this one. Little did I know when I was giving my pre-race spiel in this frigid thirty-degree town that I would end up with a personal best on this challenging and hilly course. I think what made it so surprising to me was that my previous best was set 25 states ago. I know I'm getting older, so I never really believed I'd tackle that time again. How appropriate at this time of year that all of this happened in lovely Bethlehem, Pennsylvania.

Video Transcript

Well I've had my eye on Pennsylvania for a long time. It's amazing that it's taken me 30 tries to get here. In fact, I was signed up for the Blue and the Grey down in Gettysburg a long time ago. That would have been in my first ten, but I wasn't able to make it. So here I am at number 30 in Bethlehem, Pennsylvania. This is known for Bethlehem Steel. In fact, they say that the country was forged here. They forged the steel here for the Empire State Building and the Golden Gate Bridge, among many other things. I'm pretty excited to run here in Bethlehem. It's just a picturesque setting at this industrial complex where they use to build all this steel. In fact, at the end I'm going to be right by what they call the Steel Stacks. I took some pictures yesterday and they don't them justice. They are huge and in the pictures, they just don't look huge but I'll get some pictures at the end. You know It's perfect. It's 32 degrees. This may be my second coldest start for a half marathon. I remember about a year ago I was caught in 25-degree weather in Virginia. I was not prepared. This time I'm more prepared. I know what you are thinking, "he can be taught!". Anyway, I've got to go around the corner to the start line. Then we'll end up over there at the Steel Stacks and I can maybe show that on video and see if that does them any justice. Anyway, wish me luck. I'm going to be running through some amazing historical places. This place being built in the mid-1700s. Off to the start of the race. See ya. Bye.

[Moments after the race]

Oh my gosh! I did it! I just ... I got a PR by I think about 20 seconds. This was a hard course. There were lots of hills and it wasn't till about mile 10 that I realized that I could do it. The last two miles I just ran as fast as I could. I cannot believe I PR'd on this course. How great that it happened here in Bethlehem. Here are those steel stacks that I told you about before. This is the City of Steel ... I PR'd here. Perhaps now I'm a man of steel. Maybe THE Man of Steel. Anyway, this has been fantastic. I'm so glad I finally did it. I thought I would never be able to do it. It feels good to know that you still can do it after all this time. What a great time I've had here in Pennsylvania! I'm on my way ... I'm going South today. Anyway, have a good one ... It's been fantastic.

https://youtu.be/TpcU0j186vI

VT Be a Hero Half

The Green Mountain State

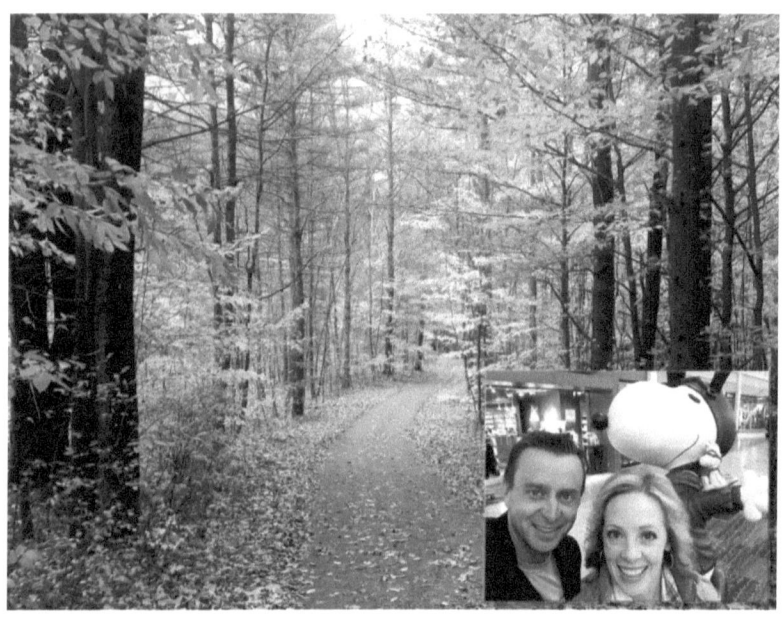

Social Media Note

Six months after crossing over briefly into this charming state on a run that started and ended in its sister state of New Hampshire, I found myself back in the enchanting state of Vermont. My wife was with me on this delightful journey through cool fall temperatures, light rain, and falling leaves on the shores of beautiful Lake Champlain.

Video Transcript

It's cold here in Burlington, Vermont. I'm super excited to be here. You know it was about six months ago when I was in New Hampshire and ran for about 8 miles in Vermont, but the race was in New Hampshire. So, Vermont, besides Utah, will be the state where I've paid for the most footfalls. This is exciting for me. Plus, I get to be back in beautiful Vermont! Even though it's kind of cold. I'm going to be running down here by Lake Champlain. This area was a strategic and vital area in the time of the revolutionary war and the war of 1812. One thing you might not know is that Lake Champlain was briefly America's sixth great lake. In 1998, Bill Clinton signed an act that made it the sixth great lake, but it was later rescinded. It's going to be beautiful, and I'm excited to go and run. The start line is right over here, and my wife is with me today. She's the one holding the camera. She's going to run the 5K. I better go chase my number. I'll see you at the end. Bye.

[Moments after the race]

What a great day in Vermont. It essentially is just a very beautiful and pleasant blustery day in Northern Vermont. In fact, I just kept thinking through the whole way, "If I had the opportunity to run in the 100-acre wood, this is what it would be like!" Running through the trails by Lake Champlain up here in Northern Vermont is just fantastic. I know that only runners get it, but when you're running through those long country roads and trails and there's a line of runners in front of you and behind you and the winds blowing and the leaves are falling ... with the rain. There's just something about it. Anyway, it makes me wish there were 50 more! Anyway, on we go. Had a great time. See you later.

https://youtu.be/78iPn6WllWY

RI COLT STATE PARK HALF
The Ocean State

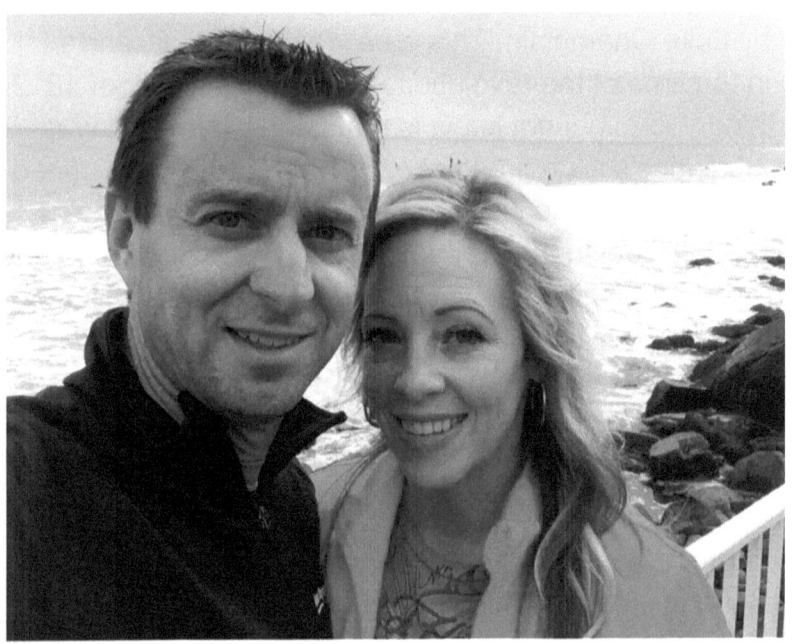

SOCIAL MEDIA NOTE

Just seven states after the largest US state, my wife and I found ourselves in the tiniest state in America. An oxymoron for sure, this delightfully petite state provided the smallest larger-than-life adventure ever. Cheers to #32 Rhode Island!

VIDEO TRANSCRIPT

It's Rhode Island, or more appropriately, The State of Rhode Island and Providence Plantations. The longest official state name in the nation which is interesting because this is the smallest state in the nation. It's the eight least populous. That means there are seven states with less people in them than Rhode Island, but what you might not know is this; it is more densely populated per square mile than any other state in the union except one. What is that state? It's New Jersey! So anyway, there are a lot of people here but you wouldn't know it today. Look at this fabulous area. We're going to move right over here. Right down here. What you have are bay views and the sea water over here. We'll be running clear around this area with scenes like this. Scenes like this with the sea air, bay everywhere. It's beautiful. There are some places here that are fun. Yesterday we went to some mansions in Newport. The Breakers Mansion and the Marble House. Just fabulous. It sure seems like the most populous area in certain places but today in Colt State Park there's plenty of elbow room. My lovely wife is running the 5K and I'll run the half. We will see you at the end.

[Moments after the race]

Wow, what a great and terrific run here in Rhode Island! We enjoyed it so much. My wife ran the 5K and I ran the half. There was a point on the track where we passed each other. So that was awesome. I think she was at about mile 3 and I was about mile 8. It was so great. You know, it's just great running around this area. You have all the different kinds of terrain. Sometimes you feel like you are back in the woods and sometimes you are running along the rocky coast watching the ocean. We westerners just envision the east coast as being this beautiful rocky area. Just fantastic. In fact, I can't even imagine being able to come here to Colt State Park and run my practice runs here. You guys are so lucky! So, I am going to declare Colt State Park a national running treasure; and the reason I can do that, you might have already guessed, is because I run this town. All right, well, have a great one. I have enjoyed Rhode Island. See you. Bye.

https://youtu.be/oKbdqixmuz0

OH CHURCHILL'S HALF
The Buckeye State

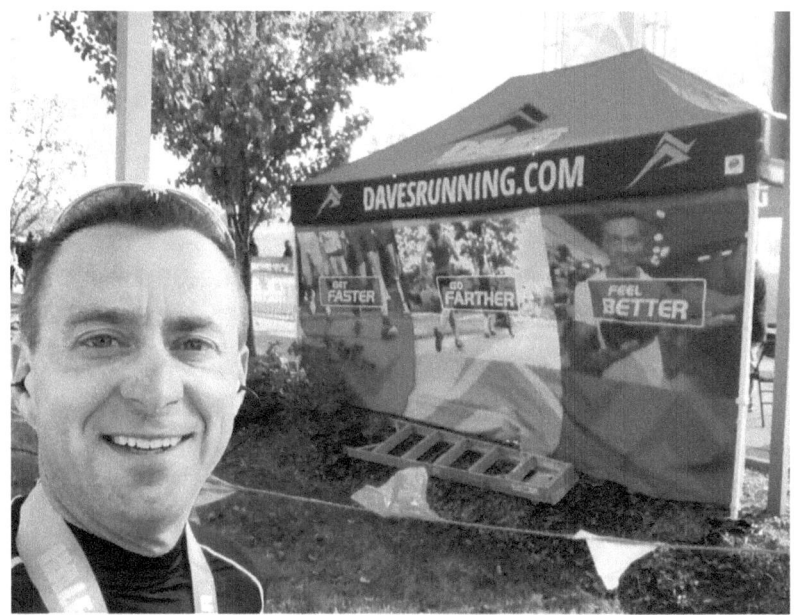

SOCIAL MEDIA NOTE

"Life is made up of meetings and partings, that is the way of it" … those wise words were spoken by Kermit the Frog in one of my very favorite Holiday movies ever. The movie is, of course, "The Muppet Christmas Carol." Kermit uttered the words in a much weightier circumstance. Still, it was hard for my heart to finally let go of the Great Lake states. How appropriate to get a personal best in my last of eight great lake bordering states. Especially when my previous best time was set the last time I ran in a Great Lakes state (Pennsylvania). Well, here's to #33 mighty Ohio!

It's a beautiful, cool morning here. I'm going to do another half marathon. I have simply loved running in these Great Lake bordering states. There are eight of them. I'm so excited because I still have one more to do but the bitter part of it is that that day is today. Here I am in Ohio just southwest of Lake Erie. In fact, we are going to run across the Maumee river which comes down from Indiana then through Toledo to Lake Erie. It was just beautiful driving past Sandusky yesterday. It's fun doing this in Toledo because that's about the most serious expletive I ever say, "Holy Toledo!" I looked that up and there are many different theories to the origins of that saying. The most intriguing one is that way back when safecrackers and the police had this understanding in Toledo that if they didn't safe-crack in Toledo they were safe. So, they would maybe pull a job in Detroit and then they would run to Toledo. To what they called, "the holy land." So thus, "Holy Toledo." So, they ran to Toledo for a little R&R and I came to Toledo to expend a lot of energy. Anyway, I'm excited. I'm going to run over to the start line now and we'll be finishing up in another location. This isn't an out and back ... that's great! We'll be finishing up at the shops at Fallen Timbers. I look forward to seeing you at the end. See you. Bye.

[Moments after the race]

Holy Toledo! I did it again! Wow, I got a PR. So, what a great place to do it. This is the last Great Lakes state that I have. The last PR that I got was the last time I ran in a Great Lakes state. I'm just so happy to be able to do this in Ohio. Wow, it's just so great. To top it off I see that they have my very favorite comfort pill after a run and it's called a Royal Red Robin burger. So, I may go over there and get me one of those but oh wow! What a fantastic race. It was hard, but I managed to

PR again. What a great send off. It hurts my heart to leave the Great Lakes but one day I'll be back, and we'll do it again. See you. Bye.

https://youtu.be/0mYG-DFSs58

NM LADY OF THE MOUNTAIN HALF

Land of Enchantment

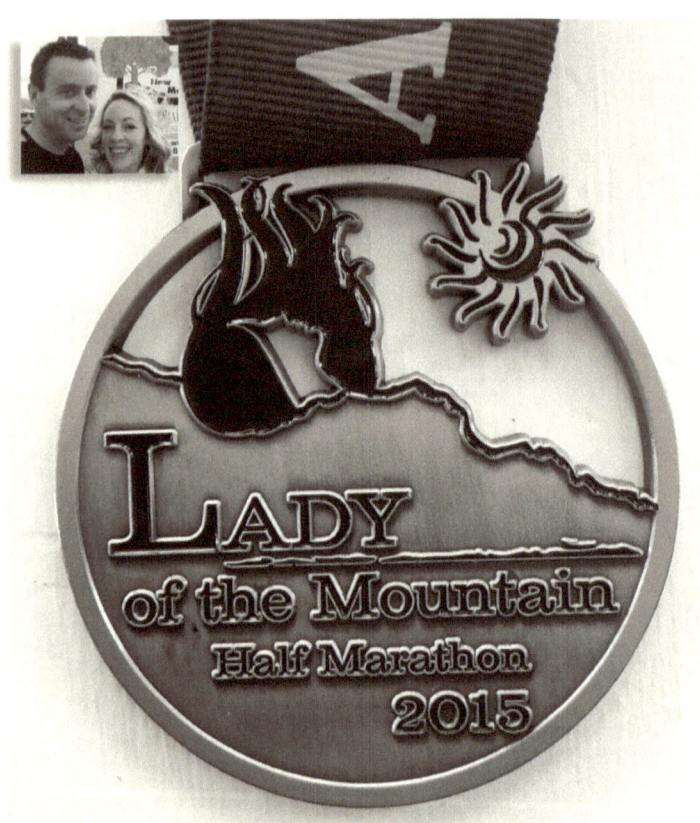

SOCIAL MEDIA NOTE

If your goal was to be abducted by aliens, what state would you choose? Well, my wife and I found out that there are much more than alien abductions in the Land of Enchantment. We found striking cactus landscapes, wonderful temperatures, and welcome quiet beauty. We'll always remember our run in the cool southern deserts of New Mexico!

Here we are in New Mexico. We had a fantastic time coming down here from Utah. We drove all the way. It's almost a thousand miles. We are almost in Texas! We are going to do a couple races on the way back and so we are excited. Through this whole experience I've had a lot of lasts and a lot of firsts. In this case I'm going to do a first. I've never done 4 states in 8 days but I'm going to do it, and this is the first one in New Mexico. The cool thing about this one is that it's probably the most mysterious one that I've got. Right behind me is the Lady of the Mountain. So that's the most mysterious sounding half marathon name I've ever had. It is amazing. They've got a little picture that I'll put on the short video afterwards that looks quite impressive. This is the land of mystery. We are a two-hour drive; about 120 miles away from Roswell, New Mexico. That's where in 1947 the UFOs stories started to come, and people started disappearing and going to outer space forever in these abductions. So, my goal in this race is to get to the end and not get abducted. I've also got my fantastic camera woman here. My wife is with me and she's going to run the 5K. We'll see you at the end. We are so excited to get New Mexico. It's beautiful here. A bit cold but it'll be perfect for running. We'll see you at the end. Bye.

[Moments after the race]

Ok, that was crazy. We knew something was strange when we came in here to New Mexico and The Lady of the Mountain. At the start of the race we were running uphill and I've never run into any wind so powerful right into my face. It was straight up. When we reached The Lady of the Mountain, we ran right up to it, and I think it was kind of a conspiracy or something. As we were running up to the turnaround point. The highest point. You could barely see, but I could tell there were less people

---

coming down than really should be coming down; but you can't really see. You're so tired and I was right by this guy with a big gap between us and anyone else. So, we were all alone. I was right behind him and we came up to the turnaround point and he touched the cone and he just disappeared! I was right behind him and I had my hand out to touch the cone too, but I couldn't pull my hand back fast enough. So, I hit the cone and ... zoom. It was like a port-key and we went inside what looked like the mountain. There was a hooded figure with a woman's voice that said, "kill the spare." This is just like Harry Potter. I'm not kidding you. I dived behind this pile of mattresses; I don't know what that's doing inside that mountain. But I'm behind a pile of mattresses and they shoot at me. It was so weird. It was just like ... what was that ... Next Generation. Picard with that woman in Insurrection where time slows down. I could see the phaser light coming at me and it was coming slow. I looked between the first and second mattresses and there was a pea-pod in it. And on the side, my good eye focusing in on it, said port-key. I reached in as the phaser fire was coming to me and grabbed that thing and ... shwoo ... I was right back where I started heading down the mountain. It was really a scary experience for me; and I know that I made it out easy because some of those guys ... I don't think they came back. Anyway, it was a great time. I just loved it because when I was coming back I did have that experience again with the time-stopping thing. With the wind blowing so bad as you're going uphill that when you're going down you are running just fast enough to be equal with the wind. So, it's turbulent all around you but yet your kind of in the eye of the tornado. Anyway, I had a great time. My wife ran the 5K. On we go to state #2 in 8 days. It's been great to have some time here by The Lady of the Mountain. See you later. Bye.

https://youtu.be/WLhqWVWTcAs

AZ Fiesta Bowl Half

The Grand Canyon State

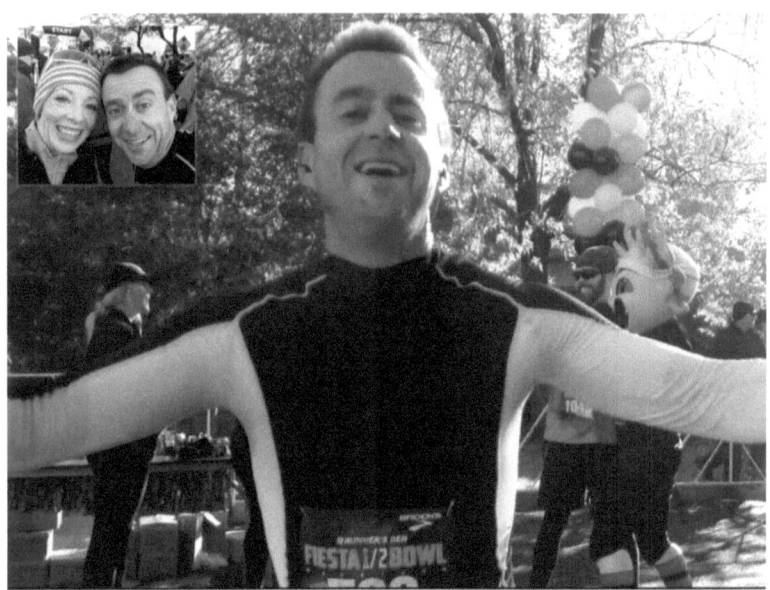

Social Media Note

Anyone else out there like college football? My wife and I sure do; so, it was a pleasure to run (my wife the 5K and me the half) during the beginnings of this year's Fiesta Bowl festivities on a sunny cold morning in the land where the Colorado River cuts a mile-deep chasm that built the mighty Grand Canyon. Kudos to amazing Arizona!

Video Transcript

This is about the latest time I've ever done a video before a race. It starts in just a couple of minutes. We're here in beautiful Arizona. You can see some of the palm trees here.

It's fabulous. It's also cool because it'll probably be the only race out of the fifty state runs that is associated with college football. Which we both love. We are excited about that. In fact, this is the Fiesta Bowl Half Marathon. Our Fighting Irish are going up against the Buckeyes here on January 1st and the festivities start today, several weeks before, with this half marathon. We look forward to seeing you at the end. See you. Bye.

[Moments after the race]

New PR! Wow! Wonderful! I just can't believe it. I've shattered my record on my second half in two days. I got 1:46 and I don't know if I will ever do that again but I'm so glad that it was right here in the west in Arizona. I love these Arizona race folks because, unlike most others, they are against hills. This was a flat course ... and fast which was good because with every mile I knew I was still in the funnel for a PR. So, it drove me on to just do the next mile as fast as I could. Anyway, we had a great time. Fortunately, we missed capturing my happy dance at the end but that's okay. What a beautiful park. We've got a long drive ahead of us, but we sure have enjoyed it here in Arizona. I'm just going to be saying "wow" in my head all the way home. See you later. Bye.

https://youtu.be/kZjeU5Uko4o

MO Run for the Ranch Half

The Show Me State

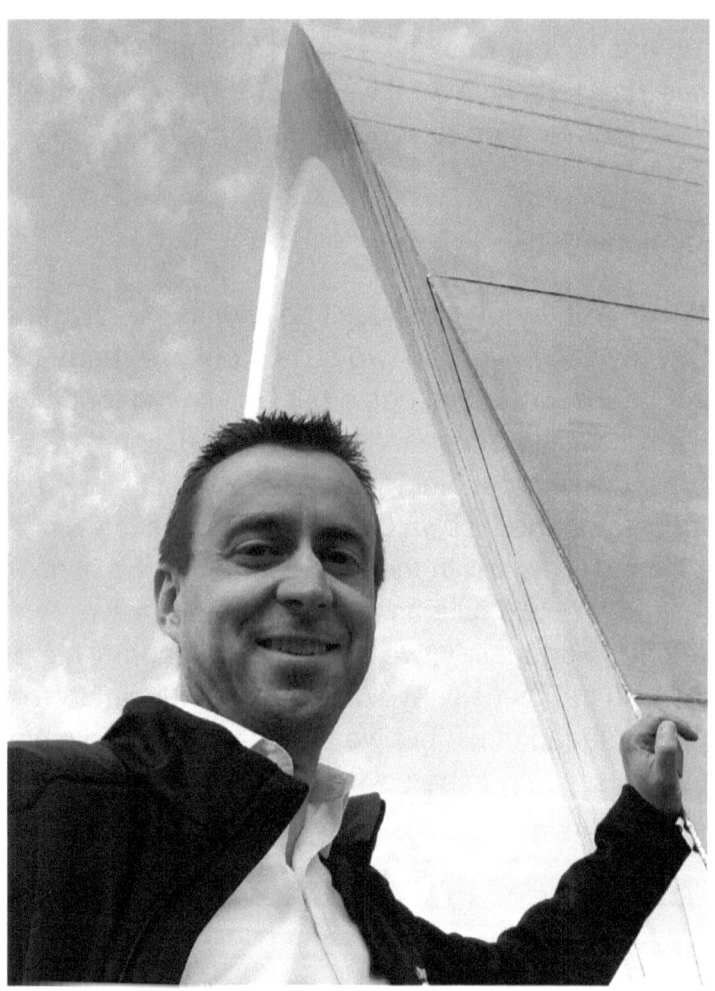

Social Media Note

Time for another cross-country drive (literally) through the Midwest City of St. Louis on my way to Springfield. Btw, anyone been to Ted Drew's Frozen Custard? Combine that with a trip to the top of St. Louis' famous Gateway Arch, and you've got the beginnings of a fantastic day. Combine that with a brisk morning run in the shadow of Springfield's university campus (where you will find Boomer the Bear) … priceless :). Chalk up another exhilarating winter run in state #36, mighty Missouri.

VIDEO TRANSCRIPT

Well, it's the mighty Missouri today. I was able to drive down through Missouri to the southwest corner from the east yesterday. It was a long drive, but it was worth it. What a beautiful day this morning. The sun is high. It's a 10am start so in 45 minutes we'll be running around this loop where all the races start at the same time on the same track; and stay on the same track the entire time. Some just do a few more laps than others. There will be 5K, 10K, half marathoners and marathoners all on the same track. That will be interesting and fun. I stopped in Saint Louis and saw the Arch. If you are in Saint Louis sometime, you need to go to Ted Drew's Frozen Custard. That stuff is good. It's where you walk up to the counter, they turn it upside down just to show you how thick it is. What a great state. Great capital. Great City. I'm not in the capital today. I'm in Springfield at Missouri State University. My race starts here in about 40 minutes. We'll talk to you at the end. See you. Bye.

[Moments after the race]

Wow … Missouri is in the books. I got a good time … I think … I need to check it out. Oh yeah, under 1:50! Pretty awesome for me. I love these races that are put on for charity and they're a loop, so they've got people all over the place cheering you on. This my 3rd state race in eight days and I need to be ready 18 hours from now when I line up at 6:30am in another state. It made me remember that when I was reading a little bit about Missouri ... evidently in 1912 the very first paratrooper jumped from a moving plane. It was a captain from the army and when he landed the press ran up to him and he said, "I will NEVER do that again." He said, "I probably did five summersaults on the way down. On the decent," he says, "I was like a crazy arrow!" So hopefully that doesn't happen to me tomorrow. The conclusion of that story is that he made his second jump just nine days later. Anyway, so I'm going to head south for #4 in 8 days and hopefully everything will work out. Missouri has been fantastic. Just a great run. See you later. Bye.

https://youtu.be/-3VYIFz2L2Q

TX WHINE NOT ANOTHER HALF
The Lone Star State

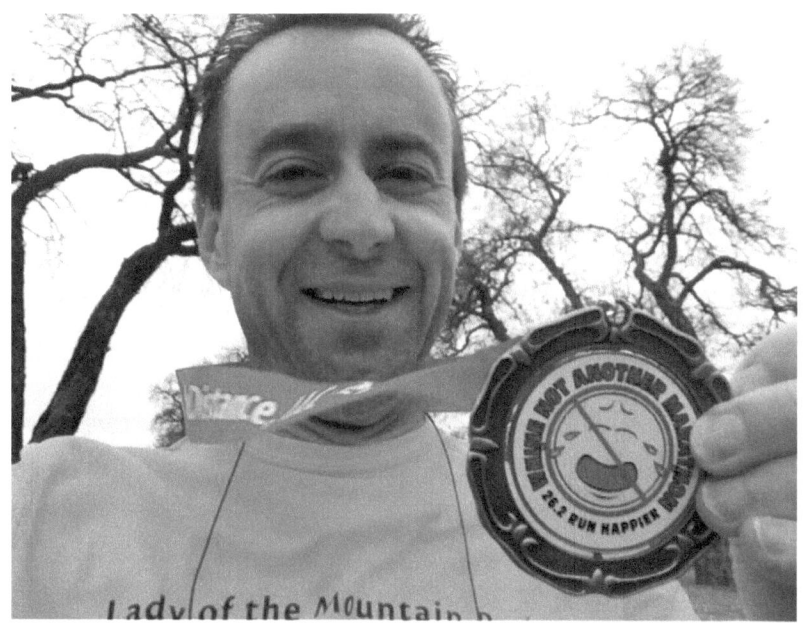

SOCIAL MEDIA NOTE

I never quite know what to expect sometimes as I move on to whatever half marathon is scheduled in the next state. Occasionally, I get something completely unexpected. As I drove into the infinite highway-spaghetti-bowls and gazillion lanes each direction in the southern metropolis of Dallas, I thought I was likely in for a hectic morning run. Not so. I gathered together with 26 other grinning runners of all shapes, sizes, and ages before dawn to start this pleasantly small event around beautiful Bachman Lake near Love Field. I've never started a race where all the runners first sang "Go Tell it on the Mountain" (yes ... I unabashedly belted it out with all the others) followed by a heartfelt prayer. I smiled at the finish line when I checked the final stats to see I had come in fourth overall (which never happens btw). Just another testament to the small town feel that provided a marvelous experience. So, cheers to my new friends in Dallas, Texas (state #37). I will never forget this unique and welcome experience.

VIDEO TRANSCRIPT

Well I'm probably not going to get another chance to do this. Wow, here I am in the great state of Texas. The biggest state in the continental United States. When you come here (I came down from Oklahoma) Texas is just a big place. As I was driving in there just seemed to be freeways going in every direction with six lanes each way. It's just crazy. But they've got us tucked away here by historic Love Field. We are going to run around Bachman Lake. We are going to start before sunrise so that's why it's so dark. When I was talking to my buddy about coming to Texas he said, "Aren't the half marathons 16 miles down there?" That got me laughing just a little bit. The half marathon here today is called, "Whine Not Another Half Marathon." Many of these people were here yesterday and ran a half marathon. What they don't know is I also ran a half marathon. I ran a race yesterday in another state and so my knees are feeling a little flaky this morning but it's going to be great running around this lake. We are going to run around four times and then after the race I will show it to you. It'll be great. Anyway, here goes Texas.

[Moments after the race]

We started early on this one. You can see the sun is not really shining through this cloud layer here at Love Field in Dallas, Texas. You can see the trail that we ran. This is Bachman Lake. I'll try to talk loud over Love Field's planes going back and forth. The event was fun because this was a Christian sponsored race and so we all met together before the race and it just had a different feel to it. Not too many people even ran this race. Probably around thirty or forty. You know that because I came in third or fourth or fifth overall (which never happens). When I was running there's a lot of older people running. There was one couple that kind of reminded me of the Odd Couple. One of them had hair down to his shoulders and they were both running bow-legged. I was coming up on them to lap them and they were running but they were going about as fast as half-walk. They were talking, and you could tell they were having a good time. As I was passing them they said, "huh, what is that? Is that the third one to pass us?" The other guy goes, "Ugh ... I thought we were in the lead." Anyway, it was just fun to see these guys. I'll go see how well I did. I did well time wise, 1:50 something. So that's pretty good for me. Anyway, kudos to these great guys who have managed to give me an experience that really has a small town feel in the middle of this bigger-than-life city. I've just had a fantastic time. Well, on to the next one. So long to Dallas, Texas.

https://youtu.be/FpbMuDmkIBA

IA   O'Round the Loch Run

The Hawkeye State

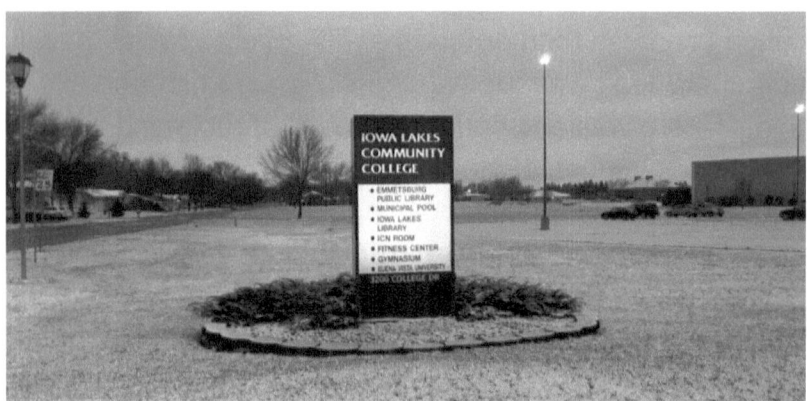

Social Media Note

Well, I finally corralled the state that enjoys the unique status of being the future birthplace of one James Tiberius Kirk, Captain of the USS Enterprise. Although I'd like to know who ordered the late-march snowstorm with more frigid, windy bite than waterskiing the Bering Strait. Still, it was satisfying to muster through the chilly winds and icy-dicey roads of America's heartland ... #38, Iowa!

Video Transcript

[In the midst of a snowstorm]

Ok ... this is one time when the internet pictures don't look at all like when you get here. Evidently there's a loch around here somewhere. We're going to go around the loch this morning. It is freezing. It's says 30 degrees but it feels more like 15. This is Iowa. Welcome to Iowa. The picture they had on the internet site had a picture of this little lake in the middle of what looked like summer. They are in the death grip of a winter storm today. In fact, I drove through the night to get here. I had just a few hours of sleep. Other than one other race I've never gone on so few hours of sleep. Going down through Minnesota it was white knuckle driving, blizzard conditions, and snow-covered roads. It's the end of March! At any rate, I love the opportunity to get Iowa. The home state of Captain Kirk. In Star Trek IV Kirk was talking to Dr. Gillian Taylor when they are at that restaurant and she says, "Let me guess, you're from outer space." He goes, "No, I'm from Iowa, I only work in outer space." I've always wondered (and the weather reminds me of this); I was reading and in some of the musicals they sing about Iowa and they say ♫ Ioway ♫. Evidently the Ioway people were a native American people that lived here (a tribe). They were called Ioway and that's where Iowa gets its name; but the meaning of it is surrounded by a bit of controversy. Evidently at one time someone came in and said Iowa Iowa Iowa and they think that meant beautiful beautiful beautiful; but there's also a variant on a French word ayuhwa that one of the other tribes maybe called the Ioway people that meant "sleepy ones." Anyway, it is so cold right now that I'm not about to fall asleep. I've even changed into the thermals that I normally don't wear but it is freezing. We'll see how I do and somewhere there's a lake. I'll talk to you after. See you. Bye.

[Moments after the race]

That was a great race, but it is weather that tests your resolve. For the first hour it was just uphill into a blizzard. Those little snowflakes are falling that sting your eyeballs. The last part of it was with the wind so that was good. It was still pretty cold and this wind bites but there's just a satisfaction that comes with doing something hard. Even though I was running down a stretch thinking if anybody saw me doing this in a blizzard they'd think I was a moron. What a great race. Sometimes you're looking at the street signs trying to apply them to you. Some of them get you down like 35 mph and you're like, "yeah, right" but then coming down here they had a few signs that said, "No Passing Zone" and so your body's like "okay ... yeah, I could do that." I caught this race on a pretty cold day, but we did go around a loch. So, there is a loch down there. So long from the great state of Iowa. What a pleasure it's been to be here in a state that epitomizes the mid-west. I'll see you on the next one. Bye.

https://youtu.be/2EFXwAYMaoc

OK Dust Bowl Series
The Sooner State

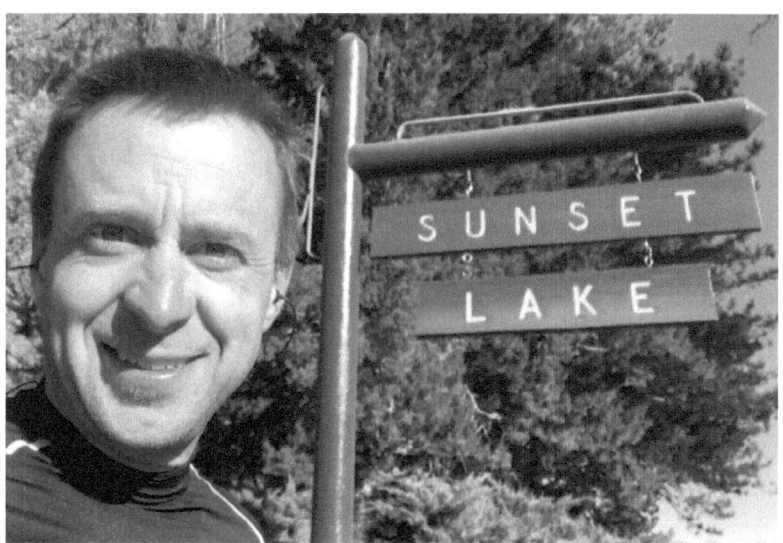

Social Media Note

In a state where the wind plays more twister per square mile than any other place in the nation, I found myself driving hours after midnight through heavy wind gusts to finally arrive in Guymon around 3am. No problem, two hours later I was up and realizing again how cold and blustery it can get in the panhandle in March. Meanwhile, just to the northwest, my wife had been turned around after many hours of treacherous driving conditions due to the unanticipated Denver snowstorm. Rotten luck for sure; it made for a lonely but lovely sunrise run on sunset lake. Only 55 folks in this one; the small-town feel made for a charming day in a delightful spot on the earth. Here's to the birth state of legendary Will Rogers, Oklahoma!

Note to self … don't sing before sunrise, you'll just embarrass yourself :).

Ok, it is cold and dark but here goes ... ♫ Oh, what a beautiful morning, oh what a beautiful day, I've got a beautiful feeling, everything's going my way. ♫ Well, here we are in beautiful Oklahoma! It took a while to get here. I think this is state #39. That's amazing. I won't even tell you about the heroics it took to get here last night. Let's just say that for the last few races I've been rolling in at 3am and then at the starting line before the sun comes up. Who doesn't love a state that has the record for the biggest pecan pie, biggest pecan cookie, and biggest pecan brownie. And, by the way, you can find a working oil well on the state capitol grounds. Pretty crazy. The race is about to start. You can see we are going to run around this lake right here. Maybe we can get some good pictures again at the end. I'm super excited to get Oklahoma. I'm up here in the panhandle of Guymon, Oklahoma. I'm really looking forward to this very brisk morning run. See you at the end. Bye.

[Moments after the race]

That was a good time for me, 1:48 considering how we got here yesterday. I must give a shout out to my lovely wife. We agreed to meet each other in Denver yesterday, and a storm came through and prevented that. In fact, she had a very scary almost-accident near Rock Springs Wyoming before the police turned her back. She drove six hours to just go home. That was tough. I was trying to fly to Denver, and all the flights were canceled. I flew from Ohio to Michigan, then tried to go to Denver to learn all flights were canceled. They rerouted me through Atlanta. Then when I got to Atlanta, the Denver flight was canceled. I called the airline and asked, "can you get me anywhere close?" The day was waning, and they finally got one seat to Oklahoma City, but I had to go back to Detroit. So anyway, I flew into Oklahoma City. I got to Oklahoma at 10pm and then drove all the way to Guymon which was a 4-5 hour drive in the middle of the night. I rolled in at 3am. Even with that, it was just a lovely race. They have their little spot of Eden here, but just a shout-out to my lovely wife. You should be here. Ok well, on to the next one. Oklahoma's in the books. It's been great. See you. Bye.

https://youtu.be/hsMS0kXEf9I

KS Dust Bowl Series
The Sunflower State

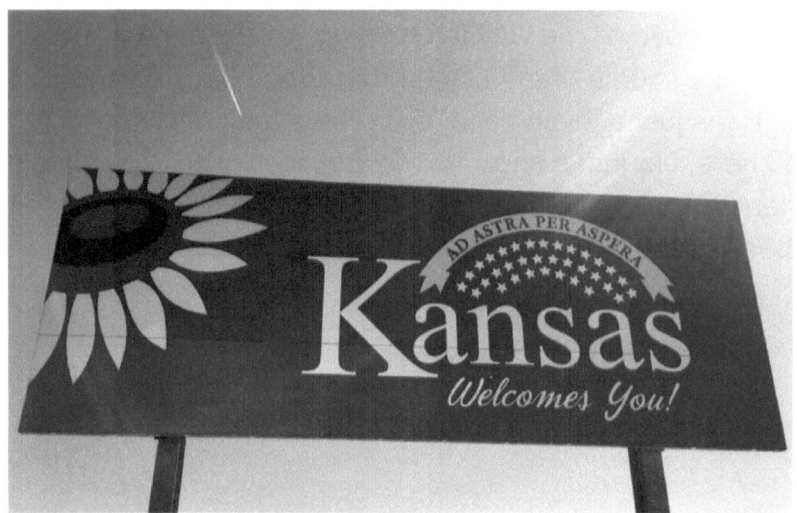

Social Media Note

As I drove across the state line, these lyrics started playing in my head, "Carry on my wayward son. There'll be peace when you are done. Lay your weary head to rest. ..." It sometimes surprises me, especially now near the last, just how much resolve it takes to keep going. To be prepared, at any time, to take advantage of any opportunity to get that next state. When I started I was so sure I would make it; now I look back and wonder how I was so undaunted, but somehow, I was. Enough of the sentimental me, I can click my heels together three times tomorrow after a fabulous race in a wonderful state. In fact, it's state #40. This is a significant milestone for me, and I've really enjoyed the friendliness and comradery in this race series. Here's to the town of Ulysses, new experiences and new friends; and I'm so glad it all happened in the great state of (did the lyrics give it away?) … Kansas!

As an aside … since we are talking about yellow brick roads. As a lay American boy, I've seen more than a few live musicals (Broadway and otherwise). Perhaps my expectations have been too high, but I've always (and I mean always) walked away somewhat disappointed and unenchanted by the experience. However, a few years ago I attended an event that was the result of a friend's suggestion. My wife was with me, and it sounded like a fun evening, so I said yes. As usual, I entered the Orlando theater not expecting much … which may be why I was so surprised … shocked really. The performance was Wicked and, to be honest, I was floored. Just before intermission when Elphaba replies to Glinda that she is no longer afraid and softly begins those melodic tones, "Something has changed within me … something is not the same"; there is a foreshadowing, in that instant, of the culmination that would raise the character quite literally off the stage in a theophany of power and feeling. When the curtain fell on the scene, and the lights came up for intermission, I was dumbstruck. Seriously, it's the only time I have been so impressed with any live show I have ever seen. Bravo, bravo, bravo!

VIDEO TRANSCRIPT

Well they need to stop holding these things so early in the morning. I'm in a beautiful place and lucky enough to be in the same state where a just over a century ago a little adventurous seven-year-old girl made a little ramp. Probably not unlike what you might use for a bicycle to do a jump. Anyway, she got a hold of her uncle who helped her put it on the top of the tool shed. So, this is an interesting uncle. She made a contraption and she took it and then went over that ramp and off the tool shed and hit the ground hard. She came out a little bruised in her little torn dress and her first words were, "Pidge," she said, "it was just like flying." You might have guessed that that was little seven-year-old Amelia Earhart who started her adventure that day. Well, my adventure starts today. I'm a excited because yesterday when I came into this state it was the first time I've ever been to the state. So that's always fun for me when I cross that line for the first time. Anyway, I'm in the great state of Kansas. So, when I put my video together and you see the picture of the sign for Kansas there. Just know that I was smiling when I took that picture. Every footfall I put in this state is a new adventure. I need to go over to the start line and take 20,000 little adventures here. I'm excited about that. Oh, one more thing before I run. I learned that Amelia Earhart, Wonder Woman of her time, shares the same birthday as me. How about that. There's only one other celebrity I know that shares the same birthday as me; and that, you may have already guessed, is Linda Carter. Anyway, I'll talk to you at the end. See you later, Bye.

[Moments after the race]

Kansas, Kansas, Kansas, loved it, loved it, loved it. What a wonderful race that we had here. We ran around Frazier Lake you see in the background. The race had a great feel. These Mainly Marathon people did a great job with the race. The only thing missing for me was a road built of yellow bricks. I guess I'm going to go find that on the way home. I've got a great day in front of me. I'm going to go conquer the Rocky Mountains in a car. My head should hit the pillow of my own bed, before 3am. So, I've got a great drive ahead of me through Denver and then up through Wyoming. Anyway, just loved it. What a terrific bunch of runners there are here, and very friendly. We'll talk to you later. Bye.

https://youtu.be/cC2aKgTQ9lc

LA Riverboat Series
The Pelican State

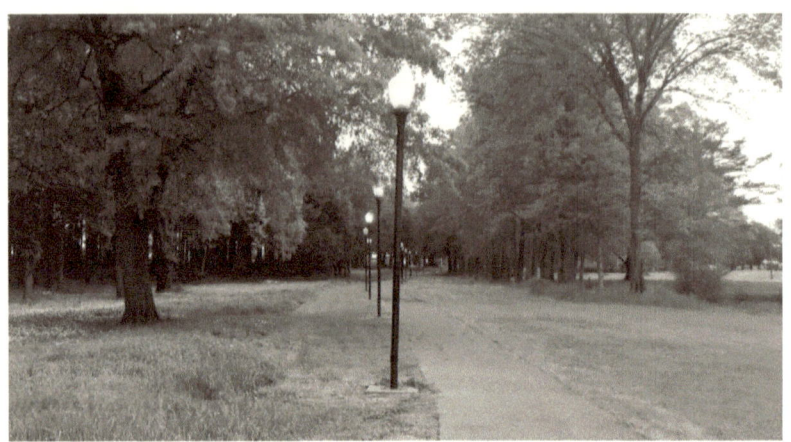

Social Media Note

I still remember, as a young junior high band lad, that a few close friends and I admired excellent trumpet players. At the time, we turned mostly to Maynard Ferguson to scratch the itch. One of my favorites is his rendition of "Over the Rainbow" (https://www.youtube.com/watch?v=ioUOZM3FyWo). Hang on to the end, the best stuff is in the last 60 seconds. Even today I still have a little Maynard Ferguson in my music library. Of course, we also admired Miles Davis and good ol' Dizzy Gillespie. Who can forget those puffy cheeks? I mention these folks to honor the best singer/trumpet player of all time, whose home-state I just earned, and who also taught the value of people and our beautiful blue planet when he shared What a Wonderful World (https://www.youtube.com/watch?v=gDrzKBF6gDU). Who else could I be talking about but the timeless Louis Armstrong and his birthplace … The Big Easy, Louisiana!

Welcome to the state that owns The Big Easy. I remember that New Orleans was probably the very first big city that I had ever visited. I was about 23 or 24. I had only been to one other state that didn't border Utah or Idaho and that was California. Then I flew into New Orleans when I was young. So that's where I got my initiation. Anyway, what I'm about to do today is not The Big Easy. In fact, it's a first for me. As I'm getting to the end of the states it's interesting that I do firsts and lasts, and this is another first for me. I've done four half marathons in eight days one other time. While I'm going to do that right now, starting with this one, I've never done three half marathons in three states in three days. Hopefully it'll be ok because I hurt my knee last night. Don't you just love this. I was coming in yesterday and it was so pretty. It reminded me, believe it or not, of my run in Montana. The only difference is wherever you step on the ground in Louisiana it seems a little squishy. This is the path I'm going to run behind me. It almost makes you want to use Professor Dumbledoor's Deluminator and get all those lights. The sun will be up in about 20 minutes. That's when we're going to start. I'm so excited to get this one. What a beautiful day! It's cloudy and 65 degrees. I'm sure it'll feel hot after about a mile, but right now it's just as pleasant as it can be. I'm so thrilled to be in Louisiana. I'll see you at the end. Bye.

[Moments after the race]

It is so beautiful here, just look around. This is what we ran through the entire time in Louisiana. What a beautiful place. It's almost surreal how beautiful it is. Well there is a series of firsts when I go through these half marathons and it took till state #41 for me to come in first place. I won the race! These Mainly Marathons are a bit smaller, so the competition is a bit lower. There was a guy on my heels the entire time. Starting about halfway through the race I could tell with every single lap he was catching up, catching up, and catching up. Finally, I was sprinting the last half mile and my right calf was going into spasms. I was just limping along, and I just barely beat him. That's great. I never thought (I'm not a fast runner) so I never thought I'd come in first place. What a great time to do it right here in this beautiful area. It just warms my heart. The state song is "Give me Louisiana" but on Wikipedia the second state song is "You are My Sunshine." What a great way to leave the great state of Louisiana. I have loved it here. We'll talk to you later. Bye.

https://youtu.be/tnpJqiyGzFs

AR Riverboat Series
The Natural State

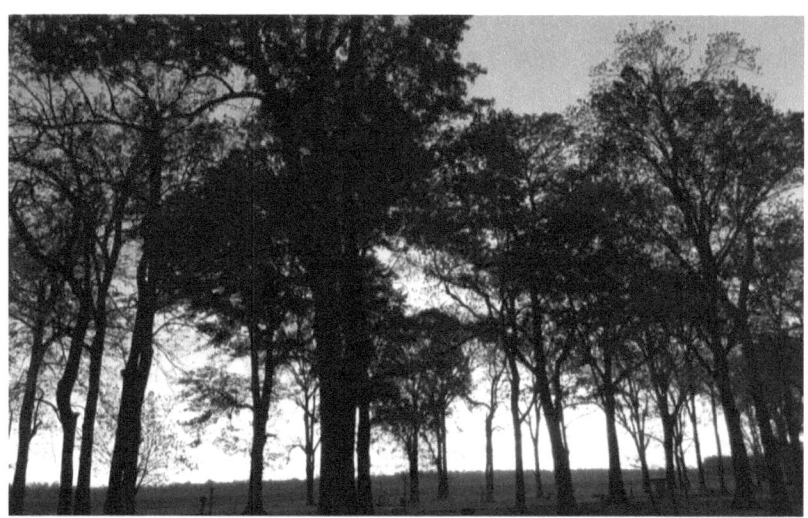

Social Media Note

A few weeks ago, I was driving through southeast Colorado across a river that bore the name of a state very far away. After arriving home, I remember asking my wife what that river was doing in Colorado. As it turns out, that river is almost 1500 miles long, originates in the Rockies, and empties into the Mississippi River. Several weeks after crossing that river near its source I got to see it where it joins the mighty Mississippi River. The state is awesome Arkansas! As an aside, several years back I started wearing black to work on Fridays, I don't know why. Anyway, now some people at work have started calling Friday Johnny Cash day. So, here's to two Arkansas sons ... The Arkansas River and Johnny Cash. Cheers!

There's no light for my face this morning. I'm here in the great state of Arkansas. They sure find terrific places to run these races. If you could see the oranges and purples in the sunrise behind me that this little digital camera is not doing justice to you would be amazed! They find fantastic places to run these races. You can see that I'm surrounded by campsites over here by Lake Chicot. I'm running the Riverboat Series and I found a story about a riverboat, and it originates right here on Lake Chicot. In the mid 1800s Lake Chicot separated Stewart Island from what is locally known here as Sunnyside Plantation. There was a bad guy and his gang, and they did all kinds of bad stuff but one of the last things they did was stole a riverboat. It was full of whiskey and they took it back to their hideout on Stewart Island and they got drunk. While they were doing that the local population went over there and wiped them out. So, we have another story where the bad guys get drunk and the good guys wipe them out. Never heard that before huh? Anyway, the riverboat sank with the whiskey. It's called Whiskey Chute. So that's an interesting story. The internet says that that spot is family friendly now, so I plan to stop by on my way out. Hopefully my chances with this race won't go down the chute. This is my second half marathon in two days and the second one [of four ... which turned out to be five] in eight days. I'm really looking forward to this run and especially this sunrise. Anyway, I'll see you at the end. I am super excited to run around Chicot Lake here in Arkansas. See you in a bit. Bye.

[Moments after the race]

Boy, you've got to love these small-town races. It looks like today we had about fifty runners running the different races. It was fun because, like yesterday, my 1:50 time was good enough to be the fastest man on the course. While in most of the races I'm at about the 25th percentile. It's been fun to "live the dream" even though it's just a fairytale really. At any rate, what a great time we've had here in Arkansas. Arkansas near Chicot Lake has been fabulous. We'll see if it affects my performance tomorrow. You know I always love it when on the second day my time is a little bit better, which it was today by about a minute. Anyway, I guess I'll talk to you tomorrow. See ya.

https://youtu.be/1DcF_FnPnuQ

MS Riverboat Series
The Magnolia State

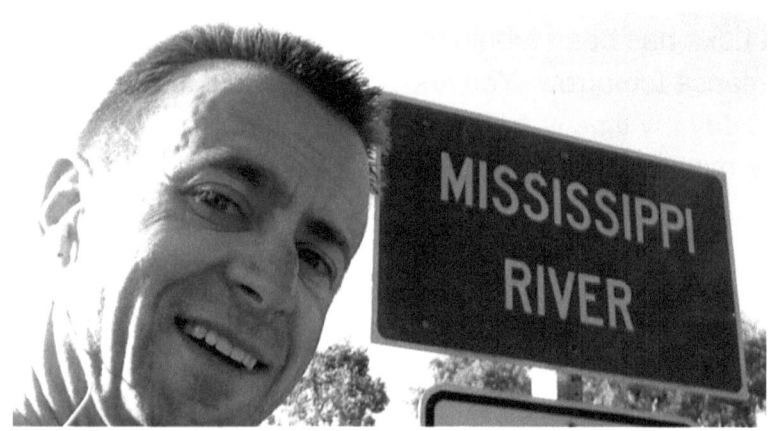

Social Media Note

I bid a fond farewell to the mighty Mississippi River and the states that enjoy its constant company. I hated finally driving away from the 2300-mile long river that has faithfully guided my many-year journey through the heart of America. In order of appearance, they were Kentucky, Tennessee, Wisconsin, Illinois, Minnesota, Missouri, Iowa, Louisiana, Arkansas, and finally #43, the great state of Mississippi. It has indeed been an experience filled with hope and wonder, but now with an unwritten future. In the spirit of Fiddler, "To Life!"

Video Transcript

The sound out here in the early morning is just something. I'm super excited to be in Mississippi. The first time I came to Mississippi I spent the day with a retired general. Every time he referred to the state he said, "The great and sovereign state of Mississippi." Of course, he was referring to the fact that Mississippi governs itself but it's got at least one more definition which is "ultimate power" and hopefully that's what I have today because this is my third half in three days. It's the first time I've ever done that. I've got one at the end of the week too, but I've never done three in a row. The other thing that pulls at my heartstrings is that I finally say goodbye to Old Man River. How fitting that I say goodbye to the Mississippi River by finally running in its shadow here in Mississippi. What a great thing. Anyway, I've got to run over to the start. Hopefully, like Old Man River, it's a good omen so today and the rest of my life I can just keep rollin' along. Talk to you at the end. Bye.

[Moments after the race]

Everybody's got their little piece of Eden and I'm just glad to be a part of it. What a way to send off the Gulf Coast and the entire Southeast for me than to be in this small series of races where I ran three in a row. On top of that I came in first place in all three. That's called a triple-double. A dual hat-trick for sure. I know that from here on out I'm going to end up back where I belong in the 25th to 30th percentile. Just a beautiful area here in Mississippi. I'm going to sign off and head to the airport. I'm done with my third in eight days, my next one is at the end of the week. I'll talk to you then. Bye.

https://youtu.be/rQ0rgqLWjy4

WV Race for Hope

The Mountain State

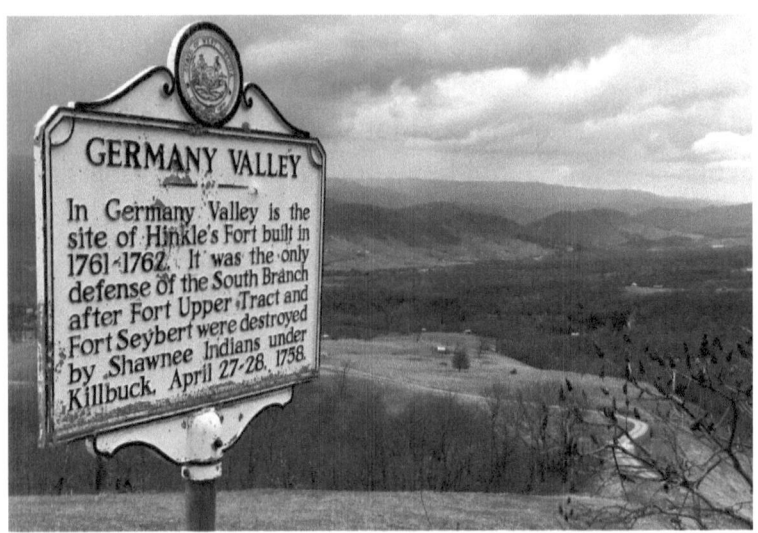

Social Media Note

Have you ever felt a connection with a particular place on the Earth? I have. In the past, I've sought these out by visiting areas where earlier generations of my family lived out their lives. In this case, however, it was not a place where my fathers once walked. After some thought, I quickly realized the connection was not associated with ancestry, but posterity. Specifically, this wonderful state once played the part of The Good Samaritan to someone I love. Many years ago, this state took two years out of her busy schedule to care for and shelter my oldest son. For this, I am thankful, proud and fortunate to have followed in my son's life-path to quietly and respectfully add footfalls of my own in the unbelievably beautiful mountains and foothills of #44 West Virginia.

Ok ... I don't know who gets to be as lucky as this. This is the state that is the unexpected journey for me. Welcome to the great state of West Virginia. I'm standing here at the base of the Appalachian (apple-lay-tion) Mountains or, if you're from this area, Appalachian (appa-latch-un) Mountains. I'm going to be running on a trail called the Allegheny Trail. It's a highland trail that follows the base of the mountains. Here's the deal; when I left my home last it was going to be the second time I would run four half marathons in eight days. I set out to do exactly that. I did three right in a row which I'd never done before and I had one scheduled for tomorrow. I went to halfmarathons.net, the bible-site for half marathons and this one in West Virginia popped up. I thought I might as well just do the sure thing. So, I drove quite far yesterday to get here. Everywhere in this country is beautiful but wow, it's just mountains and every road is in a mountain place. Can you see the misty mountains back there? There's a little bit of light rain. We're going to run a little bit late. It starts at 10am. That's about an hour from now. There's something different about West Virginia. I spent a lot of time driving in West Virginia, at least Eastern West Virginia, yesterday and it's almost like it doesn't belong in the East. It evidently has the highest average elevation as a state than anything east of the Mississippi. At first, I thought that it felt like it belongs in the West but it kind of doesn't belong there either. It is just a little treasure out here with unique and beautiful terrain. I'm so excited to line up on the starting line here and run on the Allegheny Trail. Anyway, I will talk to you at the end. See you later. Bye.

[Moments after the race]

You know, if you died and went to Heaven you couldn't find a more perfect day to run here in wonderful West Virginia. Wow, maybe one of the best runs I've ever had as far as just being pleasant. Running up on the highland trail up into the mountainside here with all the fog. Anyway, just loved it. There's a feeling here that you don't get anywhere else. I'm so glad that I ended up coming further into West Virginia than I thought I was going to next month. I feel like I experienced the real West Virginia, or at least the West Virginia I want to remember. Anyway, it looks like it's the end of my "unexpected journey" in the West Virginia misty mountains. I better run off and see if I can pick up my next packet here in six or seven hours. I will talk to you soon. West Virginia, thanks for a great race. Bye.

https://youtu.be/gnruip_Qhbw

DE Coastal Delaware Festival
The First State

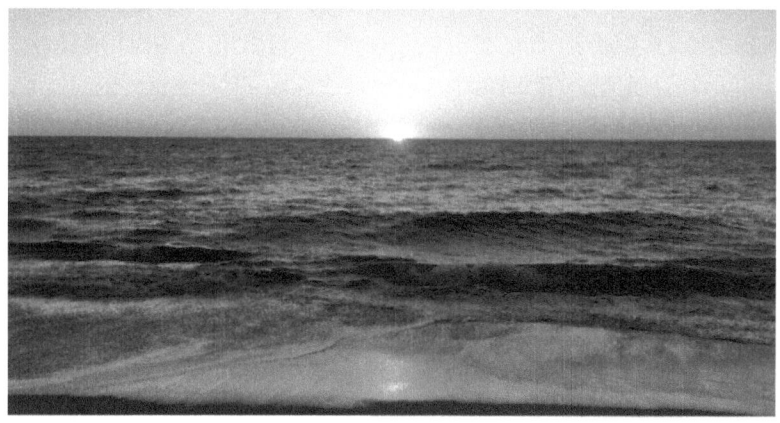

Social Media Note

I love the west, but I've always been somewhat envious of the east coasters. They get to see the sunrise before anyone else. There's just something about being present as the day's potential rises from the place where the ocean meets the sky. In this case, I got to experience that wonderful feeling on the eastern edge of America while the rest of the country still slumbered in their beds. I also admit that running this state meant a great deal to me since it was my last eastern state. The irony doesn't escape me that my last eastern state's motto is "The First State". As some might imagine, my feelings were tender on this one. So much so that I hesitated to post the video for several weeks now. Finally, last night I recorded a preamble from my backyard in Utah to help describe some of my feelings as I was finishing up that race. I can really say that as I finally drove away and boarded the plane for my home in the West, that the east didn't want to let me go.

Perhaps like Harry Potter I might ask, "Is this real? Or has this been happening inside my head." I may never know, but the eastern states will always have a special place in my heart. Like Caledonia, they call to me. Perhaps it's because this reminds me of the whole of this grand adventure and makes me really reflect about where I come from. Perhaps "that's the reason why I seem so far away today." Here's to my last eastern state, The First State … Delaware!

VIDEO TRANSCRIPT

[A few weeks after the race]

After running in 45 states so far, I admit to being teary-eyed twice after reaching the finish line. The first was #22 up in Maine. It was the first time I had ever run two races in two days and the experience had a powerful and profound effect on me at the time. The second time was this race in Delaware. Despite building all these videos, I really am a private person. I always hesitate sharing what I consider to be very personal moments. Delaware was difficult for me. It was my last state on the Atlantic coastline and my last state east of the Mississippi. It just all culminated in my head and my heart of the fulfillment of a very difficult and rewarding journey through the whole of the American East. It's a journey I will never forget. In talking to you today, I guess I just wanted the opportunity to say what I said in the video for Maine, "Thank you for sharing this private moment with me."

[Moments before the race]

Well, what do you think of when you come to Delaware? I'm shaking this morning. It's cold out here! It's about 50 degrees. You can't go any more east without leaving the shores of the United States of America. I've never been in

Delaware before. When I drove in I was surprised that before you get to the beaches it's just farmland. It's pretty. It's like you're in Iowa or something as far as the farmland. I'm all alone this morning here on the beach. You can see that I have it all to myself. My car is parked over there by the start line. I don't know what your preconceived notions are about Delaware are but for some reason the thing I think about is that Delaware is place where we bring our fallen soldiers that we send across the ocean. When bad things happen, and we bring their bodies back to their families they go to Dover Air Force Base just up the street here. So, Delaware, in my mind, is the gateway for that. A lot of families have been here to greet their loved ones as they come back from war. At any rate, I am thrilled to be here in Delaware; the last eastern state that I have. How fitting that the last state that I have on this side of the country is here by the shores of the sea. I'm excited to go and run this race. I better get over there now. We'll see you at the end. Bye.

[Moments after the race]

Here we are, back at the beginning. [a little emotional on the video] Sorry ... I have been all over the east now and I hate to see it come to an end. People of Delaware you have a great state here. You have a little bit of everything, including just a little bit of me. I bid a fond farewell to the Atlantic. What a great time I've had. I just couldn't ask for anything more. I can't wait to go back and finish this in the West. And I will finish it. Well, it's time to go.

https://youtu.be/elD9Ph7toRA

NE Half Hastings Half

The Cornhusker State

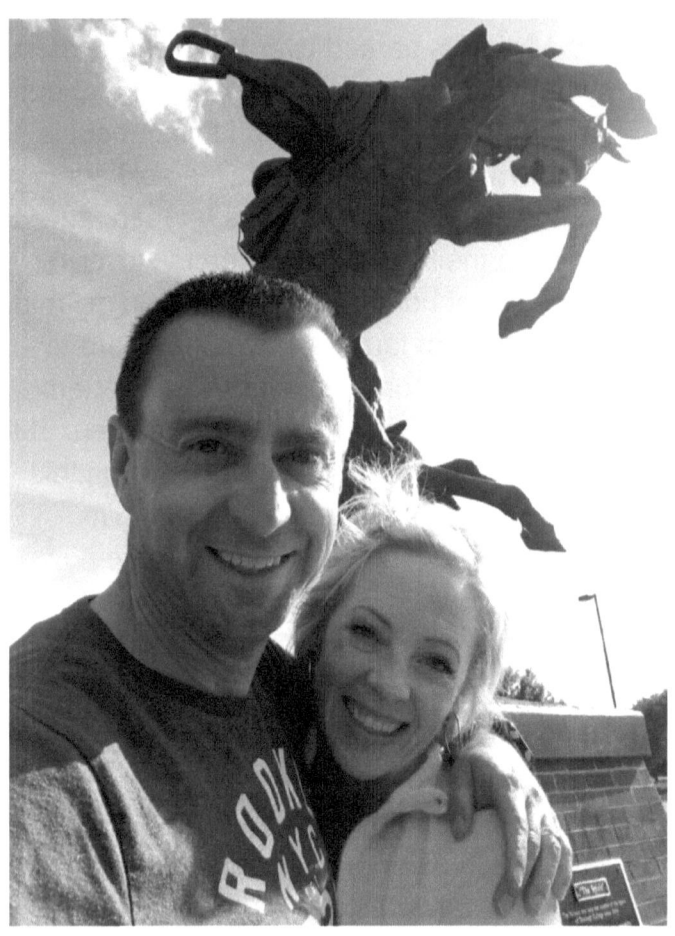

Social Media Note

My wife and I took another long road trip (we are getting pretty good at long road trips ;). This time to a pleasant little town called Hastings. It was the generosity and friendliness of the people that really impressed us in this wholesome and affable place. Incidentally, Hastings happens to be the birthplace of one Edwin Perkins. Many of you may not recognize the name, but the kid in all of us owes him a serious debt of gratitude. After all, he was the ingenious inventor of Kool-Aid! "Kool" eh? Beside that undeniable connection :), many of our ancestors walked this land on their way west which had us feeling a fond and strong connection with this beautiful place. We had a terrific time together in half marathon state #46 Nebraska! ... and then there were four.

VIDEO TRANSCRIPT

Welcome to Nebraska! You've just got to love that name. I think it's the best state name we have. I just love saying, "Nebraska." The S-K is good. Alaska is good, Nebraska, Cornhuskers ... pretty good stuff. Anyway, we drove a long way yesterday ... a long way to arrive here at Hastings. You can see the little Hastings Middle School sign right behind us. We're excited to run here. Of course, this isn't our first rodeo but I read yesterday that Buffalo Bill held his first rodeo over in North Platte just a few miles down the road in 1882. The thing that really struck me as I was looking at some of the things in Nebraska is that the most mentioned landmark as people crossed the country over the Oregon Trail is Chimney Rock. Some of my ancestors crossed the plains a long time ago and they used some of the Oregon Trail and in their diaries, they mention Chimney Rock. Here we are generations later and we are passing those same landmarks. We feel a connection with this land and we're excited to be here and do this run. The start line is right back there. My wife will be running the 5K and I'll be running the half. Just a fantastic morning. If you could feel the temperature out here, you couldn't ask for anything better. We have just loved being here in Nebraska and look forward to this run. We'll see you at the end. Bye.

[Moments after the race]

Here we are at the end. As I was running this half marathon I was thinking, "if any of you are looking for a new place to live you might choose Hastings Nebraska." This is just a beautiful place. As my wife and I have been here the people have just been fantastic. We've just been treated well here. This is as beautiful as it gets. We've ran through this park, I don't know what it's called, but there are fountains everywhere. On one of the overpasses we were running over several trains. We were high and there's just this little railing on the side and it almost makes you dizzy since you're up so high. Holy Cow ... just beautiful stuff here. Anyway, I've been very satisfied with Nebraska. We've just loved it. Nebraska, you've got a great state here and we're thrilled that we got to share it with you, even if it was just for a day. Anyway, we'll talk to you on the next one. See you. Bye.

https://youtu.be/cAVGI_0xB1w

SD DEADWOOD MICKELSON TRAIL
The Mount Rushmore State

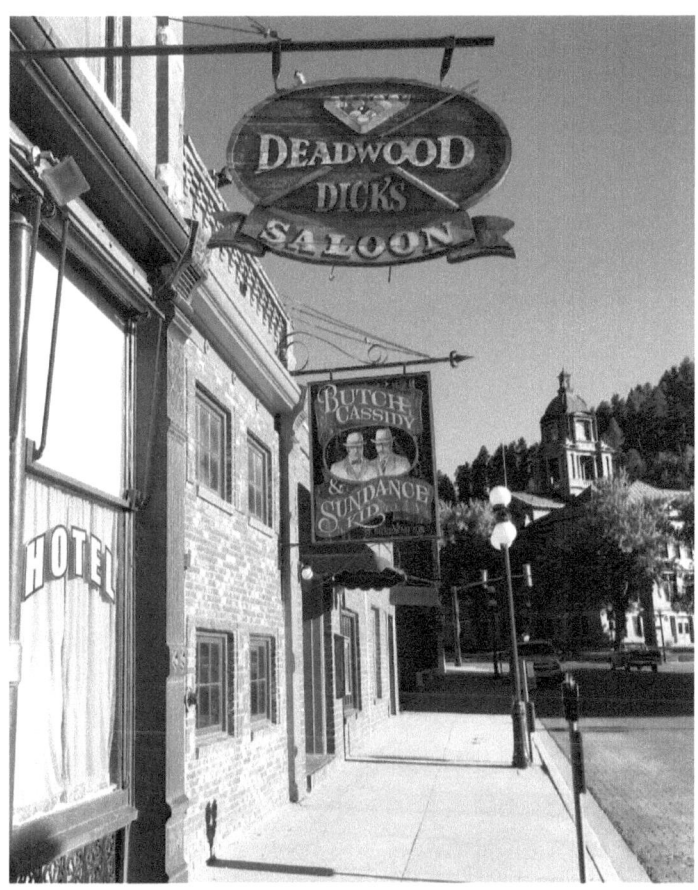

SOCIAL MEDIA NOTE

Deadwood … hmmm. It sounded interesting, so we went. As
we arrived our surroundings suddenly necked down into a
smallish v-shaped canyon. Just enough space for a tiny town;
with a small escape route on the other side up into the Black
Hills. The buildings in this town were different. They were

hotels, shops, and saloons of the old west. As we inched further into the town, we found it decorated with information about the likes of Wild Bill Hickok, Calamity Jane, and other notable western legends. As we parked and walked past "Deadwood Dick's" we finally realized we were someplace special. It was amazing to us that we made all the arrangements and arrived at this unspoiled old-west spot on the Earth before truly realizing that we were in the one-and-only town of Deadwood. We walked around admiring the enjoying structures and stories of the past. Early the next morning I was bussed to the race-start above the town in the beautiful Black Hills forests to run down the crunchy forest trails and through the crisp mountain air back to the old-west oasis of Deadwood, and #47 South Dakota! … and then there were three.

VIDEO TRANSCRIPT

Well, this half marathon was a real surprise for me. I looked it up ... South Dakota. It looked like I could drive to it. There was one that was called the Deadwood Mickelson Trail Half Marathon. I thought, "Deadwood ... that's a cool name." So, we came up here and what a surprise. It is THE Deadwood, the one they talk about in movies and have the plays about. They had Wild Bill Hickok and Calamity Jane. They are buried just up the street in Deadwood. It was like walking into the past. What a pleasure! It's just amazing to me how different all these places are. I've only had two races like this one (this one and the race in the Olympic Mountains). Here I am at the top and I'm about to head over to the start line. There are amazing views and I look so forward to running down this trail. It's a beautiful sunny morning. Down at the bottom my wife will be waiting for me. Then we'll have a few more minutes in

Deadwood before we must drive back to Logan. What a pleasure, I'm excited to start. Talk to you at the end. Bye.

[Moments after the race]

Welcome to the end of the Mickelson Trail Half Marathon! Like I said above, this was just amazingly surprising for us stepping back into the old west here in Deadwood which turned out to be THE Deadwood town that we all read about and know about. Anyway, what a great race. It was downhill most of the way. I was on a PR pace but just barely didn't make it (by about 44 seconds). One day I want to come back and run this race again. This was an fantastic race. I'm glad my wife was here with me. We've got to run back to the hotel and then drive to Logan but every state that I do I'm just so amazed by how terrific all the people are and how great the location is. Anyway, we'll talk to you on the next one. See you. Bye.

https://youtu.be/Dg6jgmzCn-E

ND Badlands Trail Run

The Peace Garden State

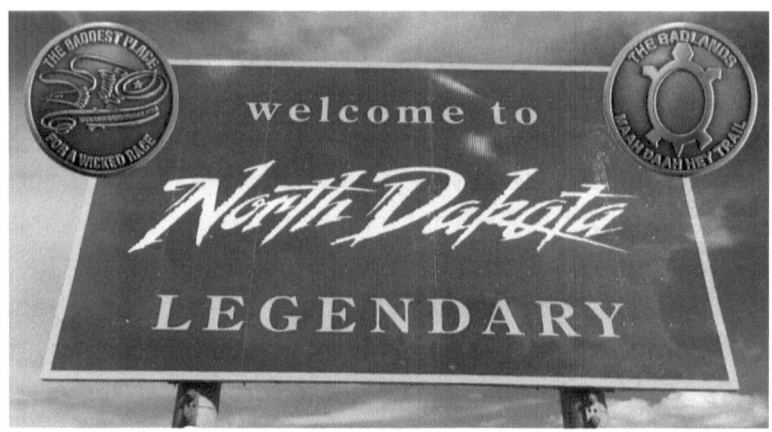

Social Media Note

A few months ago I asked a close friend about running in the infamous Badlands. A smile crawled across his face as he described the packed clay, soft clay, rocky ground and steep slopes that often characterize the rough terrain found in the heart of the American Badlands. If you ever plan to visit the Badlands just off I-94 in the heat of the summer months, fill up your gas tank, check your coolant levels, and pack plenty of water for yourself. You'll be able to enjoy Theodore Roosevelt National Park, Little Missouri National Grasslands, Watford City and the Missouri River. I was fortunate to have several family and friends with me for this race. The Badlands half marathon lived up to its name as I scored my slowest time ever on this daunting summer morning mountain run (2:24). Despite the trail difficulty, I had the time of my life in nature's wonder ... state #48 North Dakota! ... and then there were two.

Well, here we are in beautiful North Dakota! We sure drove a long way to get here yesterday. We drove all the way up through West Yellowstone Montana where we saw Seven Brides for Seven Brothers, and then we drove the rest of the way. We spent the night here in North Dakota. There's a real beauty here in North Dakota. In fact, you may not know this, and this will be the only video that I mention this in, but my wife and I celebrated our anniversary yesterday. As I was reading about North Dakota, the state flower reminded me of my wedding anniversary. The state flower is the Wild Prairie Rose. Another thing that I read about North Dakota is that it is the geographical center of the North American Continent. So, there's some Zen going on here. As I run today hopefully that'll help me out. You can see right behind our heads the start of what they call the Badlands. The Badlands run through North Dakota and South Dakota. I read a few stories about North Dakota, and several of them (at least the recorded ones) are about Theodore Roosevelt. He came up here to North Dakota (we're barely north of Theodore Roosevelt National Park). He spent time up here and evidently, he didn't mind catching criminals with his bare hands, tying them up, and taking them in. I'll let you read about that on the internet. We are excited to be here in wonderful North Dakota running through the Badlands. I've got a lot of elevation in front of me so I'm a little worried about that, but I couldn't have scripted this any better. To be up here with family and it's my last northern border state. There are a lot of runners here. I think there's about 90 runners doing all the races. We'll run over to the start and then talk to you at the end.

[Moments after the race]

That was the Badlands half, and it was pretty "bad." In fact, on a trail like this you've got to keep your arms, legs, and mostly your eyes inside the trail at all times. As I was headed back, I was thinking about what I said before about the Zen part of this place (running in the center of the North American Continent). I don't know that I've mentioned this before but when I'm running in other places where there's just farmland; you'll be running and suddenly, you'll feel like you are at one with the outside. Then you realize that your cadence is matching the sound of the irrigation sprinklers, and it's surreal. I was thinking about that as I was running up through this area listening to all the crickets and wildlife. You feel like asking yourself if this is this random noise, or is it a concert? Well, on to the next one. Bye.

https://youtu.be/ZKsJLkOusHU

NV E.T. Full Moon Midnight Half
The Silver State

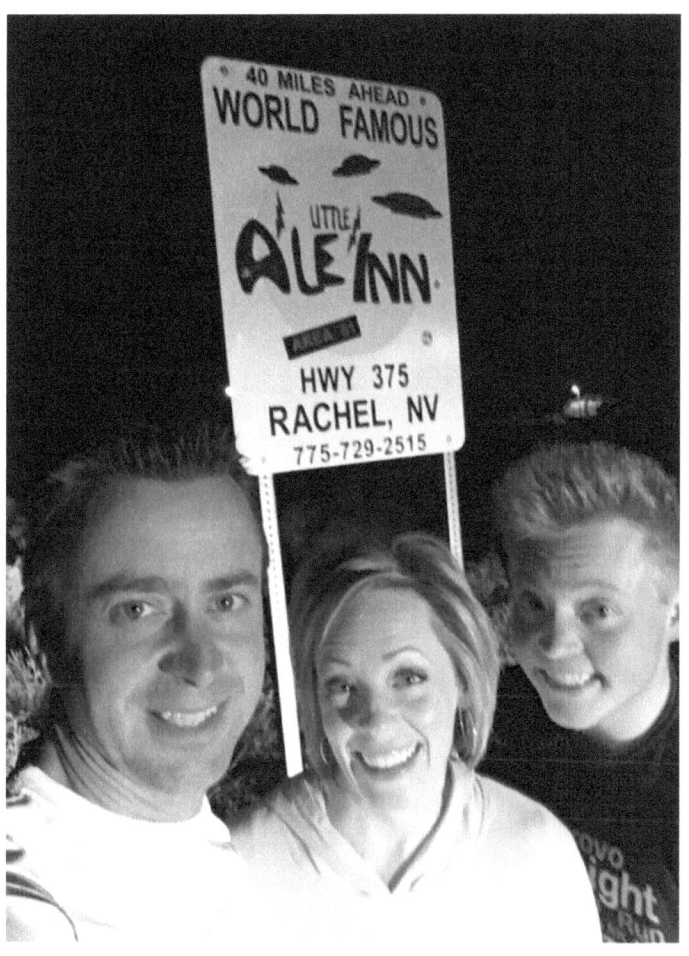

Social Media Note

Where in the world is Extraterrestrial Highway? Well, it's tucked away in a nearby desert; about an eight-hour drive from my house. Last week I drove away from northern Utah with my wife and son bound for this lonely stretch of nefarious road. We started our trek around 2pm so we'd arrive at the infamous Black Mailbox (seriously … you can google "The Black Mailbox") a few hours before the race start of 12:30am PDT (that time is not a typo!). We all knew it would be a long trip since we planned to drive to the race, run through the night along the Extraterrestrial Highway under a full moon through alien-infested "Area 51", and then immediately drive all the way home (barring any alien abductions of course). I'm happy to report that we all arrived home safely and had a fabulous experience in the state where I once spent two years of my young life … The Silver State, #49 Nevada! … and then there was one.

VIDEO TRANSCRIPT

Here we are in the middle of the night in Nevada. We are in Area 51. It's been fun as we've been running these half marathons, that every year in August the E.T. or Extra-Terrestrial Half Marathon comes around and it's always here in Nevada. It's right next to our home state and every time my son and I are deciding whether do it. Now finally at state #49 we are here in the middle of the night; we'll be running through Area 51. Amazing stuff. We're here by the famous, or infamous Black Mailbox. You can go and look it up on the internet. There are some eerie stories associated with Area 51. There have been folks who are pretty sure they have seen flying saucers. In fact, we passed a sign, and I'll include it on my video, coming here to this spot that shows flying saucers and other-worldly things. I was even reading where people were testifying that they worked on flying saucers here. We'll see. As an aside, I consider this the video I never made. My son was with me for the first three states and now we're here at state #49 and we're finally getting some video. I didn't have any video in the first three states. The starting line is just over there, and we're going to head over and start running. My wife is going to drive over to Rachel Nevada to the A'Le'Inn and wait for us. I'm super excited to finally get Nevada! A state that I've spent a lot of time in in my life. We're finally here and look forward to seeing you at the end. Bye.

[Moments before the race]

Wow. We are at the beginning of the race. We've got people here. They're all decorated in lights. This is going to be super fun. My son and I are right here. I don't know if you can see him but there he is. We've got glow sticks. We're about to run and get abducted by aliens. I better put this away. See you. Bye.

[Moments after the race]

Well we made it through. That was a long hard run, but it was delightful. As I was going through the center part of the race, the moon was very bright on the rolling hills so it looked like you were in a lunar sea. Very relaxing but I'll tell you what ... the first half of this half marathon was 4 or 5% incline and it took a lot out of me, but we just had a fabulous time. I was so glad that my son ran it with me. No one was abducted by aliens but by 3/4 of the way through, I wished that I had been abducted by aliens. Anyway, we've got a long road back but I'm so glad that we were able to come to Nevada. You guys have a just a great state here. We had a fantastic run so thanks to all the people who put organized the event. Hopefully we'll be back one day. We'll talk to you on the next one ... on the last one. See you. Bye.

https://youtu.be/sOHMPHbf1G8

OR Sunset Bay Trail Run

The Beaver State

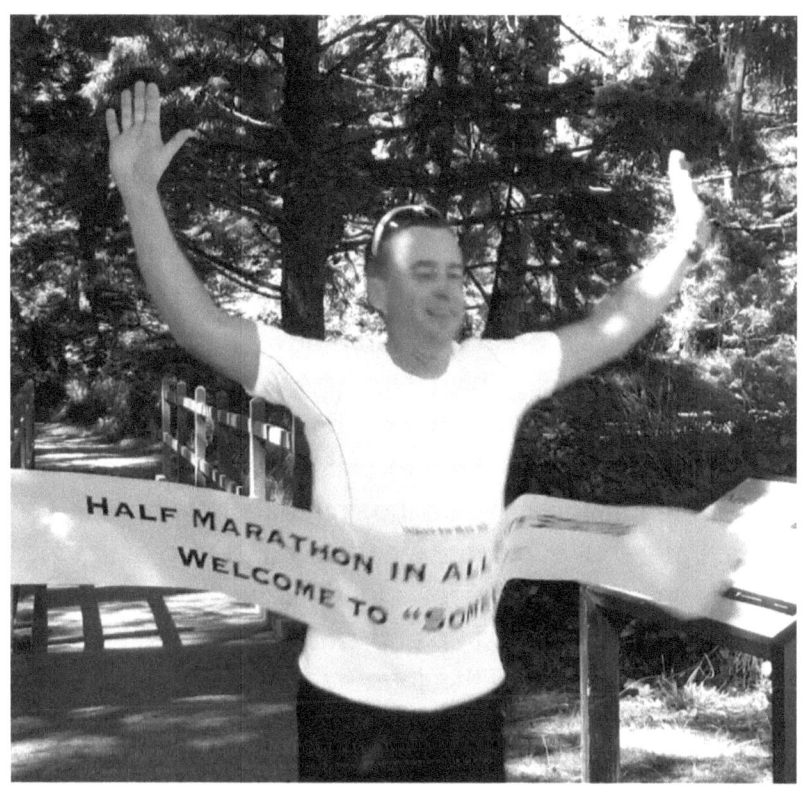

Half Marathon in all Fifty States
Welcome to "Someday"!

Social Media Note

First, hats off to my friends in Oregon who put on an amazing event. It was likely the toughest and certainly one of the most beautiful courses that I've ever experienced. As I would encounter a bend in the trail, I would think, "are you kidding me, that's the most beautiful vista I've ever seen." Then I'd round the next bend and think it again. Before and after the race, we drove almost the entire length of western Oregon and were amazed at just how distinctively beautiful it is in this wonderful state whose motto "Alis volat propriis" seems to capture the spirit of beauty and freedom that is uniquely Oregon. It means, "She Flies With Her Own Wings." As we experienced these Oregon wonders, I was feeling very mixed emotions. Have you ever worked so hard for something that you began to fear as the end suddenly approached? This was exactly what I felt as the appointed hour neared. As I raced across America early in this journey, I was so full of eagerness and faith that someday I would actually arrive at the final finish line. Midway through, the bigness of the effort started to weigh on me. I admit that I often wondered how I had once been so sure I would eventually finish. Near the end, the reality of the final finish line slowly crept into my heart as I purposely pursued the end with all the effort I could muster. Saturday morning, I tentatively crossed the final threshold here in Oregon. Later that evening, I stood on the beach of the mighty Pacific as twilight sent shadows long across the land from the West to the East. I looked up and smiled as the first evening stars signaled the end of this journey of a lifetime. I have loved this experience. The journey will find safe harbor in my memories forever.

VIDEO TRANSCRIPT

Well, here we are at the final finish line. Welcome to Oregon! Here we are; you can see the beautiful bay behind us. We sure have enjoyed the last couple of days. We've been here in Oregon, and we've been to the Umpqua River. It's just beautiful. Then we drove to Sunset Bay State Park and into Bandon (in the Old Town). It has just been fabulous. I just can't tell you how great it was or how great it's been. For my early morning walk in the mist here by the Pacific Ocean; everything seems perfect. Anyway, we're so thrilled to be here. It's just been so crazy as I've run in all the states that finally, we're here at the end. As I think back, the state where I first began to understand that this goal had an end date was probably in Ohio when I ran my last Great Lakes state. Since then I've had my last Mississippi River state, my last state in the southeast, my last state in the east, my last northern border state, and now it's my state in America. How perfect it is that I get to finish it here where every day the last rays of the setting sun hit the land; the last land in America. It's been a pleasure. Now I get to go and line up on the starting line for the last time. Anyway, we'll see you at the end. We're just thrilled that we can do this here in Sunset Bay State Park. Talk to you at the end.

[Moments after the race]

Well ... wow, I think I saved the hardest one for last! There were just shy of 2000 feet of elevation (total ascent was 1725). I ran along the beach of the Pacific Ocean. I ran along the cliffs over the Pacific Ocean and in the mountains in the forests. I just couldn't ask for anything more. We all get a handful of "Somedays" in our life, and I get to cash one in today. What a great day! I pass this milestone with a happy heart. As I think of the future, the way is clear and I know what I'm going to do tomorrow. What a great journey this has been. I'm not one for long goodbyes. We'll see you on the next adventure! See you later. Bye.

https://youtu.be/8f0kB5QqV-c

Note that the local Coos Bay newspaper wrote a nice article describing this half marathon finale (see link below).

http://theworldlink.com/sports/community/utah-man-caps-journey-at-sunset-bay/article_89973116-6e07-57c3-9d63-d91d37244060.html

Epilog

When all is recorded in the annals of history, I hope there is at least one entry of someone achieving a great and worthy goal who ascribes part of the motivation to excel to one Fifty State Runner, a regular guy from anywhere USA, who once ran a half marathon in every state. Like Charles Dickens, "I have endeavoured in this Ghostly little book, to raise the Ghost of an Idea." To remember to occasionally extend past the boundaries of comfort, physical or otherwise "which shall not put my readers out of humour with themselves, with each other, with the season, or with me. May it haunt their houses pleasantly, and no one wish to lay it."

What's next for me? I'm not sure, but don't be surprised if someday you see me running on some lonely stretch of road, somewhere on this land I love, that stretches from sea to shining sea.

ABOUT THE AUTHOR

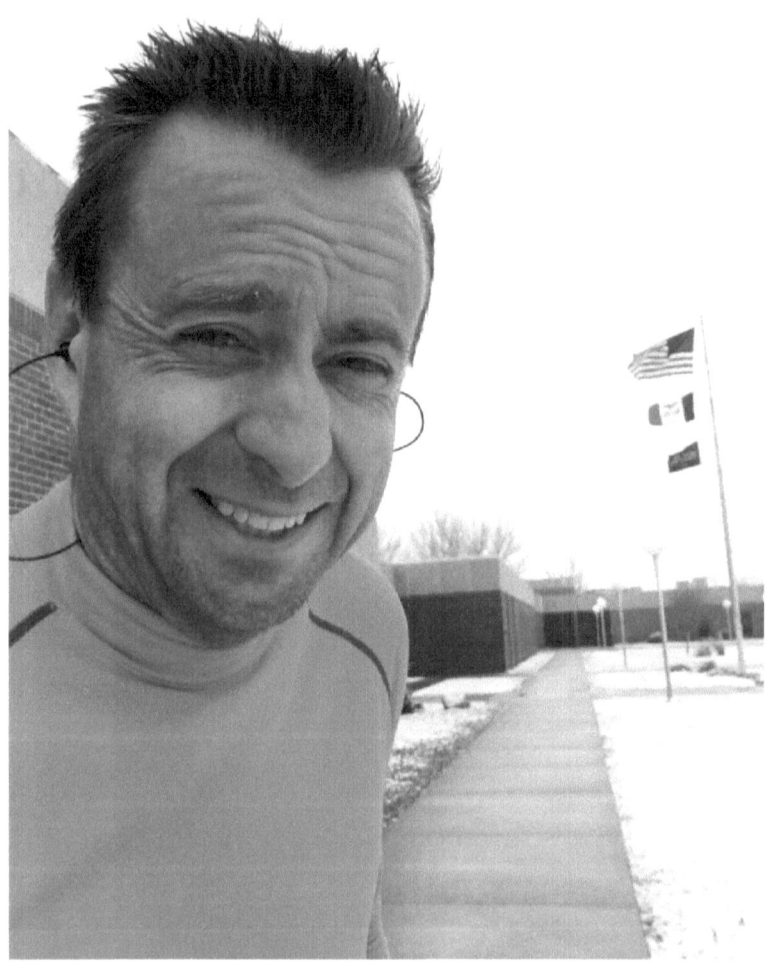

Fifty State Runner is a business professional and father of five who started running as a hobby not many years ago. He promptly lost 70 pounds as a result, but not before he ran his very first half marathon in Utah. To this day, one of his favorite parts of any race is the time leading up to the start.

After running so many events, the eagerness and nervousness still surface just before the gun sounds. He smiles as he recalls these welcome and anticipated moments.

CAN I ASK A FAVOR?

If you enjoyed this book, found it useful or otherwise, then I'd really appreciate it if you would post a short review on Amazon. I do read all the reviews personally so that I can improve future versions.

Thanks for your support!

www.ingramcontent.com/pod-product-compliance
Lightning Source LLC
Chambersburg PA
CBHW050451290526
45786CB00006B/2251